I0791659

Neuroakashic®
The Great Observer

A Neuroscience Progress

Ana Silvia Lara

BALBOA.PRESS

A DIVISION OF HAY HOUSE

This book is a work of non-fiction. Unless otherwise noted, the author and the publisher make no explicit guarantees as to the accuracy of the information contained in this book and in some cases, names of people and places have been altered to protect their privacy.

Balboa Press books may be ordered through booksellers or by contacting:

Balboa Press
A Division of Hay House
1663 Liberty Drive
Bloomington, IN 47403
www.balboapress.com
844-682-1282

Because of the dynamic nature of the Internet, any web addresses or links contained in this book may have changed since publication and may no longer be valid. The views expressed in this work are solely those of the author and do not necessarily reflect the views of the publisher, and the publisher hereby disclaims any responsibility for them.

The author of this book does not dispense medical advice or prescribe the use of any technique as a form of treatment for physical, emotional, or medical problems without the advice of a physician, either directly or indirectly. The intent of the author is only to offer information of a general nature to help you in your quest for emotional and spiritual well-being. In the event you use any of the information in this book for yourself, which is your constitutional right, the author and the publisher assume no responsibility for your actions.

Any people depicted in stock imagery provided by Getty Images are models, and such images are being used for illustrative purposes only. Certain stock imagery © Getty Images.

Print information available on the last page.

ISBN: 978-1-9822-5893-1 (sc)
ISBN: 978-1-9822-5892-4 (hc)
ISBN: 978-1-9822-5910-5 (e)

Library of Congress Control Number: 2020922874

Balboa Press rev. date: 03/03/2021

About the author:

Ana Silvia Lara

Born in the city of Comitán de Domínguez, in the state of Chiapas, Mexico; bachelor in Economics, graduated from Universidad Popular Autónoma de Puebla (UPAEP) México. Founder of Akashic School Inc and creator of Neuroakashic®. She is an author, speaker, instructor and certified coach by Secretaría de Educación (SEP) México.

In addition, it has training studies for instructors, genetics, psychosocial risk factors, SOLVE methodology, clinical certification for stress, anxiety and self-regulation, among others.

She has more than 12 years of experience sharing classes, courses, sessions, consultations and certifications in person and online, individually and in groups. For a few years from 2012-2017, she shared the traditional Akashic® training known as Akashic Records.

Starting in 2017, she began to create, develop, give, transmit and share the International Neuroakashic® certification face-to-face and online on an e-learning platform, as tools of transformation, integration and renewal, to achieve the balance of brain power, the harmonic or coherent state or Neuroakashic® potential, to children, youth and adults as practitioners and facilitators, national and international level.

Table of Contents

Thanks

This book would not have come to light without the collaboration and contribution of many people that I have met throughout life: friends, users, consultants, teachers, students, facilitators, practitioners, situations, events and circumstances that have contributed, thank you all, thanks to love and light.

In memory of my father Gustavo Lara, and in honor of my mother María Concepción Avendaño, my puppy Barni, who is a friend and companion, my other part and extension. Thanks to my cosmic parents, who made it possible to complete this book, as well as my children and my life partner. My gratitude to my sisters, nieces, to all my family and to my family network system. Thanks to my niece Paola Ramos for being part of the Spanish edition and to Paulina Serros for the English edition.

All my thanks and honor to Dr. Hamer, Dr. Jacobo Grinberg and Nikola Tesla for their legacy to humanity, thanks to the legacy that these great scientists have left us, we currently have empirical scientific evidence of the functioning of the Neuroakashic® potential balance. Thank you to all the users, practitioners and facilitators of Akashic School®. Thanks to Dr. Icela Sánchez and Dr. Jorge Flores, for their contribution and love to share.

I invite you, without judgment and expectation, to open your heart with the great master key, which is the principle of unity. Honoring and respecting are the pillars and principles of the Akashic School®, hand in hand with commitment, loyalty, responsibility, love, faith, patience, trust, certainty, discernment, word, truth and thanks.

o   This book has been edited in Spanish and translated into English.

Prologue

The intention of this book is that when you open it and start reading, each word will fill you, transport you, transmit you and expand the love and light in your heart. Finding you, recognizing the great human being full of love and light, who is already in you.

One of my greatest missions in life is to spread the word, knowledge and the principles of unity. That this book reaches homes, schools, families, offices, work, etc. and that we can share from here, expand and generate that consciousness of unity.

Read and share this book, read it from the unity consciousness point of view, from the purest love, from your cells, and that what corresponds to each one is projected in your neurons. That from the moment it is read, pure and infinite love is activated to share and expand this consciousness of unity. I take the strength of my ancestral lineage that is already in me, all those women and men who preceded me to take this to all parts of the world and expand them.

Thank you for giving and sharing this gift, remember your divine essence, we all are and come from love. Knowledge is to share and expand it to all. I have decided to share with you my mission, teaching and transmitting with the example, that of accepting and fulfilling the obligation of service and humanitarian love, and standing put the spiritual gifts and abilities that make us beings of love and light. To write a book is to transcend all the borders that exist.

My mission is to teach and transmit the essence through knowledge with love, creating and generating unity consciousness. Multiply the legacy that is already in me, in you, to humanity. What is important is what is in the heart, to give and share the teachings of love and to expand it from the heart. This book, is my graduation, is made with and from love, which it closes a cycle and opens new ones to share and expand this consciousness of unity.

Everything has a time and a cycle in our life, mine is here and now, I hope that you read this wonderful book, find the answers that you require at this moment in your life and can be the helm and directionality to execute the grace of love in your life and your environment. Knowledge is in the heart; it is opening yourself to receive the new.

My commitment to the n+1 field is to share and that this will transform your life. The light is in you, the light is in me. The light is in us! The heart only receives what it has been prepared to give and share. Open the borders of your heart to the unknown. The heart is our key that expands the legacy to other places, to be the issuer of love, is to give and share through an open and kind heart. Dare to fly from the nest, looking through the heart, observe, give, share and receive.

The true act of love is the opening of the unity consciousness, to which this tool, technique, style, philosophy of life and multiple evolutions leads us to serve humanity. Let this book be the headlight, pillar and anchor to achieve your own transformation towards the great observer, give yourself the opportunity to experience it and renew your own life. Enjoy it.

Introduction

Mental health is a very important topic today; in this book we will talk about how to live in a state of complete well-being and health, physical, emotional, mental and social. Live in balance, peace, harmony, clarity and mental performance, in a consistent and equanimous state; This is achieved through balancing brain power or performance, integrating the Neuroakashic®, as a mental health and wellness tool, to mitigate and reduce the risks of psychosocial factors such as stress, emotional and work stress, anxiety, depression, fear, anguish, trauma, among others.

According to the World Health Organization (WHO) and the International Labour Organization (ILO) 65% of employees suffer or have suffered job stress, which has a negative impact of over 80% in cases of low productivity. According to the WHO in 2020, the main cause of sick leave is stress, in addition, that stress, anxiety and depression affect our immune system and suppress immune cells.

For this reason, Neuroakashic® is an emotional and mental health containment program; it is the cellular fuel, the great observer, the consciousness of unity. This book presents Neuroakashic® as a life tool to achieve a balance of health and well-being; It is proposed as an educational, adaptable and self-sustainable model to reduce psychosocial risks.

Therefore, it is a tool within everyone's reach, in the process of expanding and awakening humanity as a whole and integrating the whole towards the great consciousness of unity. Through three axes, a virtual continuing education, Neuroakashic® program has an online modality with an E-learning platform where it shares international certification, in addition to conferences, master classes and online congresses, among others. The second axis is the creation of virtual and in person theme parks and the last axis is the creation of Neuroakashic® campuses, cities and communities, in order to share and expand.

Neuroakashic® is directed and designed for the general public, to work in children, youth, adults, groups, companies, organizations and corporations. And in various areas: educational, business, health professionals, security, and the general population, nationally and internationally; in order to achieve balanced state, well-being, productivity and thus improve our quality of life.

The aim is to have an observer in each house, increase the number of critical mass and emphasize the massive awakening of unity consciousness. Neuroakashic®, is complementary to all medical and / or psychological treatment, without any creed or religion. We transmit with honor this philosophy, tool and lifestyle.

Let us remember that in the Universal Declaration of Human Rights in its art. 1: *"All human beings are born free and equal in dignity and rights and, endowed as they are with reason and conscience, they must behave fraternally towards one another."* *Talking about dignity as principles of unity.*

Akashic School® will have fulfilled its mission, transmitting, sharing and expanding the sacred word, which is love and light. One of the missions is to give, under the principles of unity, to share and expand. We all come to evolve for the great encounter towards unity. Akashic School® is transformation, integration, change, union, unity, renewal, expansion. Love adds and is the step of our evolution; we teach, share, transmit and expand the mastery of love. Love adds, the whole adds, unity adds and it already is.

The invitation is to unite and motivate ourselves, to share and expand the path of light, love, evolution and unity consciousness. Learning is the light, and leaves the power of love to act without intervention. When you are ready to receive, this book comes to you. I invite you to open your heart to live the unmissable on this journey. I honor and thank you for trusting the light in you.

CHAPTER 1
Principles of unity

The principles of unity

> "The principles of unity are the
> pearls of the great price"
>
> Ana Silvia Lara

The principles of unity are the observer's ABC; they are the basis of creation. Neuroakashic® cellular fuels were first given and later, by balancing brain power at the hyper high level, these principles of unity came to be shared and expanded. Through these principles you understand how the universe works. These principles are something that you wear as the dress, it is not something external, it is like the dress with pearls, diamonds, crystals; and they are related to interference patterns, n+1 fields and neural network systems.

These principles of unity are unwavering, it is not about believing, it is about connecting with unity consciousness and feeling that you already are. This consciousness of love and light, of sharing, vibrating, resonating, expanding and amplifying are principles of unity, from ourselves, in our hearts, as well as that of our families and environment in general.

Build and constitute your own life under the principles of unity. It is suggested to build a life and share these principles, in a relationship, life project, marriage, family, business, company, it is suggested to work these principles or at least have the intention to participate, life and work, this will be the light, every day. It is enough with your heart intention, to give love, this will be the main fuel; You will be integrating these principles of unity, and of all the words that end in – ity – and – ness - for us it means light; read these words 3 by 3; it has a neural effect on the user. Allow, take a moment to observe and integrate between each line:

- Perdurability, Impeccability, Durability

- Totality, Multiplicity, Replicity

- Simplicity, Serenity, Severity

- Affability, Flexibility, Honesty

- Sensitivity, Integrity, Reliability

- Rationality, Credibility, Equanimity

- Unity, Reality, Grandiosity

- Oneness, Fecundity, Dignity

- Assertiveness, Fraternity, Luminosity

- Solidarity, Effectiveness, Productivity

- Sexuality, Equality, Equity

- Parity, Duality, Polarity

- Necessity, Toxicity, Natality

- Mortality, Gratuity, Sorority

- Vacuity, Permissibility, Vulnerability

- Impeccability, Affability, Eternity

- Goodness, Vulnerability, Fraternity

- Prosperity, Directionality, Continuity

- Reciprocity, Adversity, Laterality
- Happiness, Accessibility, Nationality
- Compatibility, Community, Privacy
- Mobility, Authenticity, Amenity
- Connectivity, Cognitiveness, Willfulness
- Impartiality, Flexibility, Neutrality
- Confidentiality, Adaptability, Feasibility
- Humility, Authenticity, Originality
- Causality, Singularity, Multiplicity
- Priority, Emotionality, Impulsiveness
- Neuroplasticity, Intentionality, Potentiality
- Flexibility, Comicality, Velocity
- Tonality, Temporality, Community
- Satiety, Society, Predictability
- Predictability, Possibility, Parallelity
- Relativity, Conductivity, Elasticity
- Viscosity, Inclusivity, Mobility
- Majesty, Unity, Voluntary
- Impartiality, Flexibility, Neutrality
- Confidentiality, Universality, Immunity
- Histocompatibility, Pathogenicity, Probability

- Combativity, Ineffability, Spasticity

- Gravity, Timelessness, Insubstantiality

- Vulnerability, Probability, Immunity

- Portability, Elasticity, Municipality

- Transportability, Frontality, Portability

- Alkalinity, Volatibility, Emotionality

- Radioactivity, Synchronicity, Subtlety

- Feasibility, Humanity, Normality

Observe the synchronicity in a harmonic state, subtlety allows us to observe what it is, allows us to transform ourselves and invites us to do it. These principles are applicable in our daily, professional and laboral life. In organizations, companies, businesses, groups and individuals.

Speaking of leaders of consciousness, in corporations, organizations, groups, business, etc., some principles of unity are: productivity, effectiveness, publicity, availability, accessibility, quality, facility, responsibility, competitiveness, proactivity, legality, reliability, freedom, dignity, creativity, sustainability and assertiveness.

The principle of giving and the brain

> "The pearls of great price, is
> the beginning of giving"
>
> Ana Silvia Lara

Giving is the same as receiving, giving to receive separates us, giving more causes imbalance or disharmony. It is suggested to build, give and share, allow the other to experience the light that is created, originates and is born in the act of giving and receiving only with the intention of sharing. Giving is the vehicle, motor, motive, foundation and mechanism of love.

It is not the quantity but the love, if giving is not the vehicle of love, do not wait for its return. Conditional giving does not return either "I give you because you give me", "I give because I hope it multiplied". When giving is its function, love returns multiplied. When giving is transformed into love and given through love, the magical, extraordinary, miracles arise.

The vehicle is giving, detached from results, expectations, structures, paradigms, beliefs, etc. The foundation of giving is love, and that love that begins with yourself and towards others, that love that is born in the heart and that expands. The love comes from the heart to give and share.

Let the main ingredient be love to give. May the relationship with love be established in all our acts of giving. May the waiting be multiplied by your giving, do not wait without love; wait with the total detachment of love without attachment, without pain, without expectation, without results, with nothing in return. Ask yourself, how do I see love? and see yourself if you are in an intrinsic relationship with love, realize that you are love.

Giving with your own will is love, but if it doesn't come back ask yourself what is your relationship with love. Integrate love and your giving will multiply. Giving is in you, if it does not return, the learning and teaching of love is represented in such a way, in any circumstance, event or situation so that you remember what love is. *Love is knocking on your door and needs to be seen.*

Have you ever noticed that giving confuses you?

There is no confusion, because everything is based on giving and behind love, love is giving and giving is love. It is in giving everything under, the premise of giving, it is in giving and not in the results of giving. Giving is the result of love, gratitude, rebirth, and unity. Love plus giving is fulfillment and that is the encounter with love. One of the purposes is to give and share, the cycle is complete, the reason for giving is love, which is amplified, expanded and unified in one.

In any situation you are going through, just remember to take the step and you will find love. Giving, love and you, is a trinitarian relationship, pure and intrinsic. It is suggested that you review how your relationship with love is and access the elevated concept of love. Look and see that love has always been there, to be recognized from the great observer; you give what you have in one glance.

Cycle of giving

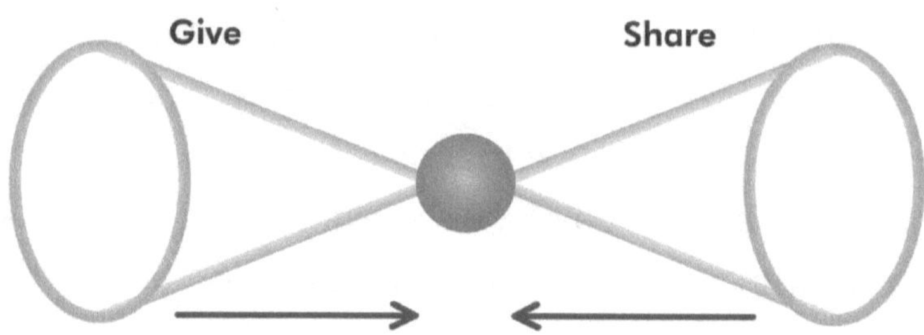

Giving is a symbiotic syntactic relationship, the ability to give is in the brain, because giving is love and is the one with brain power or Neuroakashic® potential. The giving process is connected as an energy circuit that is connected from the heart to the cerebral hemispheres and this cycle of giving can be affected by the n+1 field (it is the way to call the summation of the fields in general). The cycle of giving can affect or deplete neurons. The fuel for neurons and cells is the same giving.

The brain system is the network system, it is the great master brain connected to others in that great network connection; in other words, it is the brain connected to other brains. That is, giving is equal to brain capacity and neural capacity. Therefore, in the heart lies the love that is the greatest force that moves all network systems, and in its entirety to neural, family, planetary, universal network systems, etc.

Giving comes from the heart, from the neural networks that connect to the brain's networks. In the absence of this cycle, it breaks with the symbiotic relationship or the harmonic state or coherence. Then the ability to give, reduces the behavior of cells and neurons, added to oxidative stress and others can cause neuronal death; so, what is the key to trigger this cycle? The answer is love.

Allow yourself to activate love from your heart, feel it, deserve it and thank it, then this cycle will begin to activate. You have not failed anyone, there is no failure or error before love, they were only tests to integrate. Learning is to observe, to be aware every day and every minute of what love is.

Then there is a relationship between the brain connection, the neurons and the cells at the level of the n+1 field. The brain connection generates fullness through the brain regions, which is where the akashic® transformers and the great akashic® matrix are connected, and from there it is brought to consciousness. The process of giving is related to neural network systems, n+1 fields.

The n+1 fields corresponding to giving are: field n+1, giving + field n+1 share = field n+1 the unit. The cycle of giving is related to the brain, cerebral hemispheres, heart, intestines, coccyx, mother earth central crystal, the neural network systems, and the neurons, mother or hyper neurons in the cerebral hemispheres. The cycle of giving is related to the feminine principle, the feminine energy, the mother earth Gaia. Giving is a motor to create something more and give it continuity.

Giving when it is shown or revealed by the field and it puts events, circumstances, tests, learning to integrate and transform giving in our human relationships, on a daily basis.

Cycle of giving

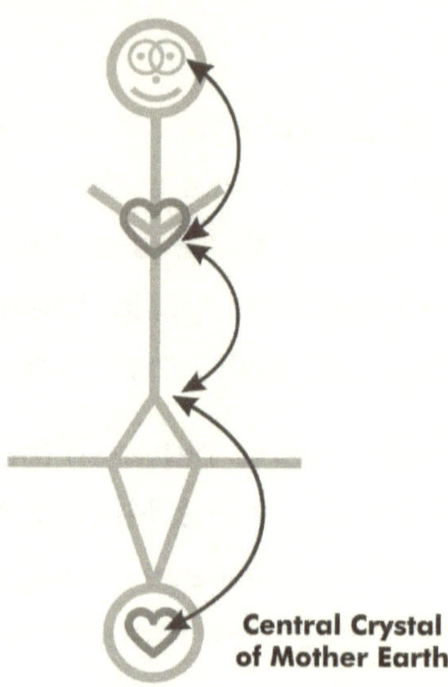

Giving and Money

Giving and the energy of money without separation is giving is receiving, giving is money, giving is gratitude, giving is the expansion of consciousness. The principle of giving is money, money is the principle of giving, money is light, it is limitless and inexhaustible as the inexhaustible source of light. If money is giving and light, it always is and already is, has been, is and will be. The energy of money has been conceived as separate from the process of giving, when it is reciprocity, that is, the energy of money is an integrative process to the consciousness of unity.

Money is the profound ability to give; is the amount of light proportional to brain power. Money depends on light, levels of rootlessness and major anchorage and the level of brain power. That is, the money is in proportion to how much light is integrated. Therefore, your relationship with money is the relationship you have with light. By talking or thinking about money, we are talking about consciousness. The energy of money activates the light processes without separation from the principle of giving. Furthermore, it activates the processes and principles of unity, seen from the cycle of giving, from the perspective of Neuroakashic®. For unity processes, it is already happening; connect from the space of love.

In the process of giving, observe how the human mind has separated money, conditions, judgments, generate expectation about it, and the principles of unity are broken. Even, it is not the amount of money, if it is more or less, but the energy that your giving takes. Observe how your giving is, what is essential and indispensable is the principle that giving has love as its vehicle, foundation, motor and motive. Are you ready to give and share?

The energy of money is integrated from giving, giving is money, money is giving, intrinsically and closely related to each other, there is no separation; talking about money is talking about giving; the process of giving is in both directions and in the environment itself. Giving in its full manifestation of love is already. Observe that giving is receiving, giving and sharing already is.

All requests in particular and in general, everything that corresponds now is in the user's network system; rest assured that whatever you require, it will be enough to commit yourself to the principles of unity and everything will be given to you, feel sustained and contained by something greater.

Transformative language

Language creates, language is vibration. The word is a code and it is a frequency. Observe how the word is anchored to the field, the greater the Neuroakashic® potential, the more possibility and probability of positively anchoring the n+1 field; therefore, it is materialized from thought, from the word and through the field, which defines the high or hyper high potential Neuroakashic®, because it works in transforming language through neural networks, having a modulating effect, anchoring the field n+1.

Language is the controlled response of the brain, towards the development of global consciousness or unity consciousness. You are conscious of your word and thought and you potentiate through transformative, overall and inclusive language. A thought or an emotion also affects the structure of the great akashic® matrix and great network systems.

The purpose is to achieve the intention, word and thought to connect them to the heart, and in this way, empower, amplify and expand from love. Therefore, it is suggested to observe your verbal and mental thoughts, since only with thought can you move the network systems. This transforming language is one in which we observe how we conduct ourselves with our own intention of the truth, that is, with the clear intention from our hearts.

As we conduct ourselves with our truth, we are connecting with the purest intention of light. Therefore, the importance of the acts of the observer and the overall or inclusive language of light, it occurs as you observe your language, and the way you are accessing your n+1 field; observing how energy moves through verbal and/or sound language. Similarly, it is replicated in other n+1 fields, this is manifested and executed in other network systems. Therefore, a sound wave or thought, word can break other chains and/or network systems.

Day by day we are in constant testing and learning, our job is to observe and that begins with ourselves; stop judging us, criticizing us, giving up doubt and confusion, stop self-demanding and self-sabotaging us. Observe it, understand it, thank it and continue. Dialogue, speech and communication is a form of contention. The value of life is one, the only safe place is love. Find it and take refuge in it, it already is.

Reflect yourself in love, look at it, feel it and project it in harmony in our hearts. Where there is harmony, there is love, that's the way it is in your heart and in our hearts. The light has a purpose and it is you, that your light invites others. I invite you to this challenge of love, to work on the principles of unity, I invite you to work every day, the transforming language, this language that goes from our thoughts, words, called the language of creation through letters or codes.

Observe how the transformation of the power of language already is; the way of communicating and interrelating with the environment is dynamic, loving, renewing, in a coherent, continuous, progressive process. Here are some examples: if a thought or word reaches you, transform it orally or intentionally before *I am love, and it is already in me, love is already in me,* and so on.

In conclusion, it is important to observe and write our

experiences and experiences, every day at dawn, thank and love everything. Love is already everywhere, in the act of giving without judging and without justifying, that is true *giving*. Giving is receiving and sharing in its maximum power and the universe responds. To realize that you are one with the whole. You are the whole, the universe colludes to be there, in the whole; you are there, you are the whole, like the great consciousness of unity.

Love

Love adds, it is the helm and the directionality. Love simply is already; it is the engine of the brain and giving is the fuel. Love does not need to be expressed or demonstrated, when it already is, it does not need explanation or justification. It would cease to be love at the time of any demand. The invitation is to remain willing to open ourselves to give love in each and every one of its manifestations. It is surrender, it is the closing of cycles and it is integration. This love n+1 field, is related to: the n+1 field the relationship with love, n+1 field relationship with the couple and n+1 field relationship of being in a couple.

Love is the divine seed and the pearl of the great price. It is the maximum power of being; love vibrates, feels and lives. Love is the step of our evolution, is the bridge to transformation and beyond the bridge, there is no reason to choose, just take the path -of love.

Love is not separate from you, everything is love, it does not need rules, nor sacrifices would stop being love; love is the purest essence and is energy. Love can be confused sometimes, possessing has nothing to do with love. Love is energy, it is not decided, it simply is.

The human being acts as he is, we are only spectators. *"Let them go into the storm"*, in other words, intervening will not lessen the lesson or learning of others. That too is love, love in its maximum power, be the observer without judgment, without expectation and let go, let be, let come.

Love breaks paradigms, forced structures overtime and in the history of humanity, it comes out of any structured and forced context into the subtle, natural, emblematic, sublime, omnipresent and magnificent. Integrate love, feel and let the feeling of love be in your heart, from the integration of love, from the beginning of giving. See love in unity, unity is love, love is you, the environment is love, love is the environment, love is you.

See how love manifests itself today in you and in your environment. The heartbeat, as a sign of life, harmonizing heart, receiving love already is. Today is the time to give yourself, love you, observe you. The moment to see us is to see the environment. Movements that are integrated from acceptance and love. Without having to decide for this or that, let something bigger accommodate and adjust. "You cannot compel anyone", compel will take us away from love.

Striving to love and be loved would also drive us away. We cannot compel or force anyone to abandon their resistances and open their arms to give or receive a hug, and move on to the next even when they don't know it. And although he has lived in heartbreak, also behind this was love. Love has always been there, even if you haven't seen it. Our daily task is to open our hearts and strengthen the infinite love that is in our hearts, let the light manifest and execute the cycle of giving.

See how the feeling of being imprisoned by some topic, person or situation is transformed. Give it to love, and let something bigger set, accommodate, and reward your actions. Stop giving power to someone else, remember that integrating is love and love is integrating. Saying goodbye is also love. Love manifests and expresses itself in many ways. Love in all its forms, and all its possibilities acting.

In the form of manifesting it is already love, *the position of the act of giving enlarges the spirit and connects it to the whole.* The power and ability to transform the perspective of love is in your hands. Everything is fine, everything is full of peace and love, the light guides, transforms and accompanies. When everyone leaves, there is light and love in you, manifesting the evolution of man.

Allow the heart to sing and everything around you to expand with love. What you do and come to do now is the love poured out and expanded in you and in others. Your essence is you, nobody can take or take away something that is sublime omnipresent. No one can take anything from you, because your foundation is the love that is within you, and it already is.

Observe through the observer without reacting, it only acts with tolerance and compassion towards the environment. Choose to walk with people who are open-hearted, who share, and decide to evolve; that vibrate in respect, love, communication, etc. *Decide, ponder, act and execute.*

Love is free, only with the conscious choice to give joy, love is the path that we all walk in each moment of gratitude. Love already is, if there is disappointment it is because there really was never love and it is appropriate to integrate into this moment; to feel that it was always love and that love was still in chaos. In your life are the people who have to be there, remember that learning from every human experience is love.

The understanding of the limiting only exists in the human mind; Deliver everything that separates you from love. Our limited perception of love is what makes us believe that it is gone or never was. Therefore, the definition of integrating is to live the experience of true love. That is the encounter with you, the realization that you have a relationship with love.

To close the circle or to close the cycle, is to access our own inner peace, that is where the cycle closes, and nothing else will be necessary because everything is destined to occur. The closing and opening of new cycles is integrated together with communication and assertiveness. Observe, without reacting, rather act, and observe that peace, calm and tranquility that you already are. Love comes when you allow your soul to be at peace, and give life to the love that is already inside and outside of you, achieving the harmonic state.

Allow yourself to the manifestation of love and of all that in itself contains, sustains and provides. Love for itself will cover all our needs, without the need for attracting love, because love is already at the cellular level. Recognize the deep love that is in you, that is the great task, and recognize that it was never outside or separated from you. It is integrated into all the realities and relativities of the great universal mind.

Light is also integrated from the root or origin, by the need to be accepted or loved. Remember to release all certainty that the couple will not come to an end, love is what gives life, and the only real thing that exists. Any human relationship that is not based on love, will lose your confidence and commitment to yourself; the answer above all is: observe that love already is.

Integrate judging, criticizing, self-punishing, etc. Observe how love is the congruence of your acts, and give yourself the permission to observe and integrate the act of forgiving, that the fight or battle was only a perception of the mind, it has never existed. It was just a wrong perception of the act of love; you are there to "give love", which is born in the energy of the heart, from the cell as a cyclical sequence of the expansion of love.

In order to expand the energy of love from the heart, allow yourself to go encounter. That is what we come to do as humanity, as a group of families, as groups, couples, communities, we are one with love. Love is energy and we have never been separated from it. The foundation or objective is to land with the energy of *love*, since we all go through the foundation or transformation process, not only physically, but at all levels in which it adjusts and integrates.

Although it is not perceived in a tangible way, something bigger is accommodating and executing in the networks. Seeing love in the person, situation or circumstance means that nothing and no one can hinder love from reaching your life because love is you. The padlocks or limits that could have been perceived by the human mind, is what we have believed or assumed there has been; Today you become aware that there are no limits to generate that level of consciousness.

Surrendering to love, consists in letting something bigger act, in this case the light; surrender to this light of love or lovelessness, give it up and empty yourself. Surrendering also means giving me permission to lose myself, to find myself again; I find my own light that is already in me. Sometimes, it is done more when nothing is done from the perspective of the observer, it lets be, as it is, deliver, accept and thank. Our mission is to give love, we are here to give love.

If a test comes to you, it is because it can be overcome with love and from love. Love transforms everything, only humility of heart can connect with the great akashic® matrix. We will have to take us to the extreme of humility, to connect with the great akashic® matrix. Now, times have changed and evolved into continuous states of the brain, which is in the process of evolving to let something bigger adjust and balance the heart within the integration process. Humility already is.

Why do some situations from the past come back to life? Because they need to remind you of what love is, intrinsic love based on unity. Love from your cells, love as energy without separation from yourself. You are love and love is you. There is no separation, one is the definition of the other, you are the definition of love, I am the definition of love. The teaching and learning about love, we all have to live it.

Behind any situation, event, conflict or war, love is waiting for you, waiting to be seen. For this reason, it is recommended not to intervene in the process of third parties, since the ideal is that each human being has his own learning to find love. If you reject love, you will have tests and lessons to learn, until you find yourself. There must be proof for you to realize love, or in what other way love would come another, if it will knock on your door.

Derived from it, the way in which love arrives and is established, is through recognition and purity, the relationship between them. Just as between love, you and the pure will, in the pure recognition of the existence of love based on the consciousness of unity. For a moment, look at the love in front of you and say: I have never lost you, you have always been with me, you are me and I am you. I take you by the hand and we are one. Do not reject love, it is probably there waiting for you to see it, it is waiting to be seen, in any way, shape or form, it will be there behind any event or situation.

Love is waiting to be seen, it is waiting for you to realize that it is there and that it has always been there for you. That you and love have never been separated and asks you: why do you insist on seeing separation where there is not? Lack is the step to see love, give yourself the opportunity and you will find yourself, you will find the being that is already abundant unlimited. We are ourselves responsible for executing that love. Our maximum lesson is to learn love.

You are the bridge for the recognition of love, the act is the execution of the teaching of love. Every day we live acts of love, every day there is the path of giving and love; just allow yourself to see it, observe it and receive it in your heart. After having lived life experiences, years later you understand what your mission was, and your mission was to create consciousness of unity and the pure existence of love. The plan was executed along with the teaching and purpose of love.

The premise of executed love and the power of love is in your hands. Love and compassion is your medicine, it is the missing link. Love for others, more than words are acts of love, is allowing yourself to be vulnerable and open to love. Now that you know what love is and the principle of giving, you will understand that we are the presence of love in our hearts and that all we are and have is that. Open your heart to allow yourself to be followed by something greater.

One attracts in his correspondence, the time has come to recognize the present moment and treasure what is being lived today, without it being a burden. Your priority is still you, work in your heart, where your power lies. Your answer is your roots and what connects to them. Without obligating or forcing anyone to give, open your arms to give or receive a hug, and remember that we are not the ones to judge these acts.

Let and allow these to happen, to manifest in your daily life. You don't need to know anything else, you don't need to know the whys, when or where, you just need to open your heart, give and share, trust the same light that is already in your heart. When there is no longer anything to forgive, our mission will be to understand that we had to find ourselves.

Understand it with love and gratitude, it is time to open ourselves to the consciousness of giving under the principles of unity, and even in times of chaos, love is there, even if we do not see it. Only ask that love and truth be manifested; the transformation of love is already. You are virtue, acknowledge and accept love, stop demanding of yourself, release the demand on yourself, stop feeling imprisoned for having to choose or for making some decision. Allow yourself to experience and live life without demands on both yourself and others.

Make the connection and reconciliation with the energy of love, this is done through Neuroakashic®, and the connection with the divine couple from the respective network systems. This reconciliation is done from the heart, experiencing the certainty that it already is, and the couple meets you. Under the principles of unity, feel the full and balanced union from your inner being, now nothing is separate.

Experience love as pure energy and connect your feminine or masculine energy with the sacred. Stop forcing yourself to want to change things, and watch this moment, accept it and let something bigger adjust and accommodate. Accept and live what is, love as you already know it. The time for the observer has come. Stop carrying or feeling that you carry something that apparently is not.

It often happens that things are not as they seem and that you are suddenly disappointed, but notice that everything is falling into place. Allow yourself to see the light in other people and allow yourself to see the light in you. Accept things as they are and do things when the motive is love. Understanding is moving forward and understanding that there is no separation, the perfect complement and the perfect partner, it is already in you.

If love were defined without prejudice, the process would yield to love and well-being, the process of anchoring and integrating love and from love. The power lies in you and it is already in you. Work in your heart, the ability to connect with people from your heart, the long wait is integrated.

You are the fertility and the life, the encoder and the bio decoder of light, just allow yourself to observe; you are evolution and coevolution, you are water, life and sustenance. There is no obstacle for being in love, as a couple and having a family, since there is no separation between love and you. You and the couple are already one with the whole; to integrate is to accept that everything is already. If in the process there is nothing more to give and share, the cycle of light has been completed.

Let us open our hearts and strengthen infinite love every day, let the light manifest and execute the laws of *giving*. That is our great teaching, to see love in manifestation of the truth, keeping the mind open to the unlimited. Find a reason and make it last, integrate your magnificent power because the consciousness of the spirit consecrates your existence.

Find yourself and you will realize what you were created for. Like two drops of water, their meeting has been integrated from other times, today they meet to take the next step of learning, evolution and transformation, together walking as a couple, as a family, as a community. That the only reason is love, if you do something with the expectation that it will be or will work, you will continue to have tests until you observe integration.

Stop forcing and waiting, see how things from the past are integrated. Forgiveness, gives you the freedom to continue, congruence is based on pure love; it only requires the engine of love. Love your fellow as our humanity, from this perspective, observe the value of life from here and of love, which is now in full existence. The love network is creating and generating bridges of respect, trust, solidarity and communication, in order to generate change as a family, as groups, as a community and as humanity.

Open your heart and let the extraordinary and magical happen. No one can judge the actions of others, because love put them there to learn the lesson. Everything has been created for a purpose, let things happen, there is no wasted time, only learning and this learning is light. Everything is a choice for the spirit. Observe how the feeling of seeing separation where there is only love is transformed. Love cannot hide. Seeing the light in him, enveloping in love, allowing seeing the light in him, will help to raise the vibration and expand the love in the couple. Connect with true love and the certainty that love already is, and that will set us free.

After sharing an endless number of lives together, we meet again to make this union and be connected for several years, decades or centuries; this union without time and space, the couple may or may not be together, in the end they are and sooner or later they will be. Therefore, generosity, brotherhood, transformation, beauty, expansion, revelation, love, compassion and goodness are integrated. Love is the one that gives life to every relationship, begins to feel that true love has never been separated from you.

Love comes to you when you stop asking, even if you don't see it, it's there. Allow yourself to feel calm, allowing the manifestation of unlimited love in what it contains. Your life partner comes when you observe and integrate the love that is inside and outside of you. Integrate any expectations and trust in the existence of love. Integrate the experience of living true love, it is your limited perception of love that makes you believe that it is gone or that it never was or could not be, when it was always love, it still is and will continue to be.

We are complete, we lack nothing. Couples love has always been there for you, receive what you have given and, in other words, don't be willing to receive less than you could give. Hand over the couple if it corresponds to let it go, the golden rule is: *it is what corresponds, it corresponds what it is.* Love does not have to be demonstrated or justified, love simply is, from the origin of nature and from the principles of human unity, the couple is conceived, anchored and materialized.

It is important to observe how it transits from the spiritual and unlimited plane and materialize it on the physical plane. In conclusion, realize from the observer that love is impersonal within an implicit transformation of light, for what it already is. Observe how everything that did not result in a timeline is resolved in an expeditious way, allow yourself to live your emotions immensely and intensely in balance and fullness from the gaze of the light.

Integrate the non-separation

> "You cannot live from the past, because the past belongs to you, nothing is separate from you, neither the past nor the future. Balance and chaos, everything is one".

> Ana Silvia Lara.

Acknowledge yourself, accept and reconnect with your original essence, connecting with your heart, allowing you to integrate the principles of unity in your daily life. Allow yourself to embrace and be embraced by something greater, love. Remember that you have the ability to integrate all disharmony in love. And even when there is pain or suffering behind it, there is an immense and great love. The learning is that you are the love you seek outside.

Integrate the situation in which you have to choose yourself, since you are the love you are looking for. Listen to your heart and choose yourself, the answer you are looking for will be presented with the truth. Recognize yourself as the divine expression of love, integrate the tests that allow us to find ourselves, you are responsible for what happens to you; allow yourself to integrate what corresponds to you and observe that internal part of you.

Remember everything is already love. Without judging, deliver all the expectations of love and allow love to manifest in your life. Give yourself permission to be exclusively with you, with your home and with your heart. Everything else can wait. Give yourself permission to connect with your inner peace and with the feeling of fulfillment. The encounter with yourself, recover your original innocence, recognize in yourself the greatness, gratitude and love at this moment in your life.

Observe that the understanding and wisdom are integrated for the understanding of reality. When you realize that behind that pain or suffering, there was also great love, one of the principles of unity is fulfilled, which is the integration of the whole; when you understand that there was no longer anything to forgive, because the forgiveness in the end has already been executed and the understanding and wisdom are being integrated, for acceptance and integration to the whole and recognition during the process. The result is to integrate in total acceptance and approval.

Integrate the whole, that which you have not allowed yourself to see throughout this existence and others. Reach your own origin, your own roots and reconnect to your original essence, recognizing yourself as the whole, and accepting yourself as you are, with your gifts, abilities, potentials and talents. Integrate yourself, embrace yourself and regain your own personal power.

Accepting yourself as you are, trust, heal your heart, and keep your faith, that your faith is bigger than a rock. To return to the origin is to integrate the past, with a message of love, and you realize that there was nothing to forgive, forgiveness is intrinsically the light itself. Go back to everything and -as your origin belongs to everything-, find yourself and you will find that it is everything, magnificence and magnified omnipresence.

The consciousness of the spirit consecrates your existence, returns to everything and is the birth of light and love from your heart, which expands in both directions inside and outside, in affirmation and confirmation. Find a point of reference in life, and there you will find the answers you have so much sought. Thank the fact of existing.

The universe knows everything, it recognizes everything, it is so wise and immeasurable, so great and majestic in its entirety. In its great majesty, love was and has been there, from all time and all lines and cycles of time, so exhilarating and so subtle. Nature is harmonious and happy, to the rhythm of the heart. Glorious and eternal gaze through your eyes; the wait is over, I am the one, I am with the one, the one and I are the same.

Connected all in the same network, we perceive the whole as one. The great gaze in front of you, unison in responding to everything required, to everything commensurable and immeasurable. From nothing to everything, from the eternity of eternities; unique and great universe. Everything is connected, past, present and future, everything is unique.

This means that in uniqueness they are one, the past, present, future and all realities. Your origin belongs to the whole, there has never been separation. The origin is yourself in all realities, time-space, and the origin is inversely related to yourself. From the connection with the great cosmos with the great life, from and to the $n+1$ field as the beginning of life, hence it goes to the blood, the plasma, the corpus callosum and the cerebral hemispheres. From the macro, to the micro and vice versa; towards the whole.

Life and death, one

> "Death is the communion with light."
>
> Ana Silvia Lara.

It is surrender to something greater. The definition of death for light is that there is no separation, we are one with everything, life is death and death is life, death and life is one, life and death is the same, live to die, die to live in one. Death is returning to the great akashic® matrix, to the network system where there is no separation. Death is flying on over the network systems; life, death and eternity, one. Eternity for us is light.

To die is to live, to live is to die; we are in constant movement and rebirth; dying in life and being reborn again, are the rebirths of the heart, it is surrender to something greater, in the corresponding and respective network systems. Our heart holds the absolute truth of love and our capacity to love is infinite. Surrender to love itself, learn and integrate forgiveness. Insist and live in the present, and it will stay by your side. It is as if time stopped in *non-time* and the principles of unity were executed.

Living is the light, but also dying is, is to be the light, to become it. You will see me in the other, you will see the other in me. Love is the only thing that exists, we are the emissaries of light. Free yourself from all questioning, it is the moment of redemption in our own light. Integrate the meaning and definition of death, as the principle of unity, under the principle of eternity, accept it, integrate it and take it in your heart. Death is life and life is the cycle that is fulfilled, death-life-death-life and so on in the cycle on time lines.

Life and death, as the beginning and end. The nostalgia of knowing that it is the end, is integrated as the beginning is the end and the end is the beginning, there is no separation. Living in the past is not living, live what is today, what the day has for you, note that you only have this day and so at the end of the day observe, thank and continue the next day. Wanting to control tomorrow is to stop living. Day by day, step by step, live and enjoy the principles of unity that are shown and revealed.

We have been taught that every act deserves a reward; the reward is the gift and the gift the reward without separation. That is, the rewards and gifts are one and they already are; there are no challenges or small or big tests, in the end everything is without separation.

Health and sickness

The human being has been conceived separately from health, as a perception of the human mind and the purpose is to integrate it through the balance that allows it to have a better quality of life. By achieving balance in your Neuroakashic® level of consciousness, you will be able to acquire that lifestyle in fullness, peace, tranquility, prosperity, healing, etc.

You will realize that these diseases at some point in your n+1 field connected with reality and that is where the disease has not been separated from health and life itself; then we can say that disease is health and health is disease. You will come to the point where you will realize that you are free, in fullness, in health, in kindness, unity and uniqueness. In conclusion, it is the way to balance and achieve that optimal state of health that already is without separation.

As Master Hamer would say: *"Illness is a special or intelligent program of nature"*, its mission is to show you that it is not separate from you and that it is the health manifested in you. So, through Neuroakashic® cellular fuels, brain power, harmonic and consistent state is balanced in users.

Integrate necessity

Necessity has a neural effect, if necessity is a function of suffering, or if necessity causes or motivates suffering. An example would be the desire, longing, need for something, for example: want to eat ice cream, what would happen? This is achieved by itself through the process of integrating the balance of Neuroakashic® potential.

The need to eat ice cream could be postponed, in the sense of the human mind's perception, and if we allow ourselves to observe how it is transformed, without forcing or trying to control, it frees us from the need to satisfy needs. Thus, liberation is achieved and the brain integrates it as a neural effect, thus achieving self-awareness. Then, the need has a deeper meaning than what we have been taught or that we have lived, that is the knowledge of unity.

Integrate expectations and judgments

"Free by the free word."

Belisario Domínguez.

We will have to free ourselves and stop judging others for their condition of giving, stop looking for pleasure elsewhere, leave the waiting and the expectation, they would be opportunities to observe, under the principles of unity. Stop looking for what is already in us, in other people. When you choose to believe in some expectations and you choose to believe something different, for good or not, in the end an expectation is created and generated.

It is suggested to stay in the acts of the observer, even from the great observer, and allow yourself to integrate all needs. As you abandon yourself and integrate the sense of feeling and living, the most present need is in you. Deliver any expectations and judgment, there is nothing that love itself cannot destroy, love, humility and forgiveness makes you invulnerable, first of all. Deliver the expectation and wait.

To judge is to stop seeing you, allow yourself to abandon yourself in love itself. Feel and live love without judgment. Only love exists, without judging anything. "The doors of heaven open and everything begins to be perceived in love and beyond love when miracles happen in your life." You do not need to judge or know, we would be generating expectations, just deliver expectation and control.

Deliver everything, there is nothing else to know, everything is already in you; trusting love is trusting ourselves. Denying love is denying ourselves, our own existence. In learning there is love, the more we observe the integration of the need to love, the closer we get to ourselves, the more we will be integrating the principles of unity.

Integrate all conditioning, integrate renunciation and total detachment. Love is not love when it is conditioned; to mention some examples: "if I give you this because you are going to give me the other, I want to know if you are going to give me so I give you, I give hoping to receive multiplied, I give more so that they recognize it, etc". It is not a matter of conditioning anyone to close cycles, but of expanding love from our hearts, under the principles of unity.

Also, stop conditioning the loved one, and the people around us. Free from all judgment, analysis, comparison, need, attachment, pain, suffering; because everything is integrated in love. There is no separation. Allow yourself to observe without judging yourself, in the chaos, in the suffering, in the pain, in everything that the human mind has perceived, and since everything is, love is there, only through non-physical eyes and a kind heart, you will be able to see it and recognize yourself.

When you realize that there is no end, that in the end there is always a beginning, that everything is part of the whole, and nothing is also everything. When you integrate all expectations, you will achieve the unimaginable, the unexpected. How to free ourselves from judgments and expectations? Through the great observer, the one who is the consciousness of unity. Keep harmony in your heart and remember that where harmony is, there is love.

The brain integrates realities, in the integrating and balancing process of the neural network system. Situations or events are reflected in the n+1 field, despite being from other realities, the balance in the process of giving is integrated from the great observer; observing the synchronicity and/or the replicity that exist in the n+1 fields in the great network system. List the first five things of your day, and examine yourself from which emotion you are being the observer. See how you see yourself.

Judgment, expectations, and criticisms of one's opinion are integrated into the whole, into uniqueness, into oneness. The question or questioning is adjusted, integrated. Go and observe from something bigger. Knowing that something bigger is working, even when we don't see it physically, is knowing that something bigger is working in us.

Integrate duality

This perception of duality is a non-existent reality, it is the one that shows us the inability of our senses to see that the person, situation or event has never left, or we have never lost them. Although our physical eyes cannot see it, everything is in perfect peace. From the light, all is, everything is, everything already is, in fullness, so close to you and so close to love.

For the principles of unity, discordances, blockages, fears, negative energy, the nature of entities or discordant energies are integrated as perception of the human mind. It integrates and does not separate, it integrates everything that the human mind has perceived as separate, or as good or bad, duality, polarity, discordance, blockages, etc.

We do not humanely eliminate these discrepancies as we have been led to believe, who is in charge of accommodating, adjusting, equilibrating, balancing, restoring the network systems is the great observer. Our mission is to observe how you integrate from the great observer, remembering that you are the purest extract of love and everything else let it go.

You are the first and the last cause in the love relationship. If something makes you believe that these disagreements have kept you disconnected from you, watch how it integrates even after chaos, wars, pain or suffering, there is great love, love has been there, although we have not seen it, it has always been there. It is time for you to meet again.

Neuroakashic®, will help you connect with the love that has always been within you, being the great observer and allowing you to observe how something bigger makes the adjustment, restructures, equilibrates and balances the respective network system. The message is to transmit love. That every moment and instant we transmit, feel and expand love, through our word, our observation, our actions, our accompaniment, our company, our smile, our warmth, our compassion, our giving. Ask yourself: what are you willing to do to change the course of your life? Where do you find love? Everywhere, so you are love.

Uniqueness

Uniting thought with the heart is the energy of love, if we just open up and allow ourselves to see beyond, where separation does not exist, where there is only union in vibration and resonance and resonance from our soul, heart, mind and spirit, expanding to others, in community, family, ancestral lineage, cities, countries, planet, mother earth, flora and fauna. See the whole without separation.

The aim is that we can perceive beyond our physical eyes the power of love and uniqueness, of feeling and living the union as a vibration, not as a word, expanding the union towards the horizon and beyond. If only we stopped perceiving ourselves as separate; stop perceiving away from love and partner, because it is already in us.

Let us allow ourselves and open ourselves to feel and perceive the whole, the union in all its definitions and manifestations. Everything is so perfect for love. Reality works as a time timer, depending on time-space. Evolve or repeat? That is the question. The lack of contemplation of reality has an impact on the neuronal brain, and an implication on network systems, has a relationship with the sympathetic and parasympathetic brain. Their relationship is symbiotic and inverse, related to the great network system.

The purpose is to observe yourself from the great observer, to encounter, accept and integrate duality and what love is. The union is reality and reality is freedom, although freedom has not been well understood, even having everything, you could feel like a prisoner of yourself, so freedom has not been defined in relation to the possession of things or money that will give you freedom.

Freedom is something inherent in every human being, it is present day by day without separation, we are born free, we live free and we die free. Integrate the belief of feeling that you are not free or do not possess freedom, because you already are. Feel the freedom, the certainty, the trust they already have in you. That which you long for is what separates you, because the human mind has perceived it as separate, then that which you long for is already, and is love.

The union from you, towards the environment already is, the union between towns already is, the union between countries already is, the union between worlds great powers already is, the union of the planet and mother earth already is, the uniqueness to everything is already, without separation.

Fullness, equilibrium and faith

Faith is a state of being that comprises the whole. The fullness is to find oneself and is to find love. Equilibrium is considered as the whole. This theory only shows what is there, shows what is happening, what is the purpose of being in equilibrium? If I am in equilibrium, I reflect equilibrium in my field, what I am reflects in my field. My connection with myself is reflected and interrelated with the n+1 fields, connecting with the great central network system, activating and connecting with the whole, with unicity.

When you meet with you there is nothing else, there is no other feeling than fullness, and the moment you meet yourself, it is the moment when that precise moment arrives, where everything is liberation, everything is already transformation, everything is love, everything is fullness, everything is. And there is nothing else, that you could not feel that was different from love, to what you already are, that encounter with yourself has always been, from all moments, from all existence, in the lines of time, has always been like that.

Even for the human mind everything is already. That fusion of mind, body, soul, spirit already is, everything is light, everything is love, everything is fullness, everything is already. Fullness is the encounter where everything already is and nothing is lacking; where everything happens and is given at the same time, from a great transformation, from this full liberation from this encounter with you, nothing is missing, everything is complete, everything is everything, everything and everything is already in you.

Concluding, you only live on love while, this in its essential and fundamental part, is you. Fullness is no longer the act of liberation; it comes from the act of full liberation. When you accept that it is already in you, that everything is in you, in that recognition and rebirth of you, fullness is in all its definitions and nothing is missing, you lack nothing. The light and all that you are is one, it is already in its entirety.

Expansion of being

How the universe is expanding, we also are it? The expansion effect is a normal effect of the universe; For Stephen Hawking, the expansion of the universe is accelerating, even at an increasing rate. There is talk of an expansion of time in the $n+1$ fields, which invites us to observe from the great observer, what happens in the present moment and integrate it.

There is a relationship between the expansion of being and the expansion of the universe, of the network systems that are part of and are ourselves. By integrating the expansion of being; Observe and stop waiting for things to happen, or expect something from people, from our environment, because it is already without separation.

In the integration process, something that does not correspond cannot happen or occur, what happens or occurs is what it is and corresponds, in order to observe without separation and let something great act, that is where the magical, miraculous, wonderful happens. Observe from the expansion of your heart to that person or people, circumstance or event, love is in them and from the environment from the outside to the heart, love already is.

In both directions, love already is. Feel content, supported by something bigger, which is love itself. Stop waiting or generating expectation and become the one with the great observer.

Acceptance and gratitude

There is no denying human nature, because there is also love. Recognize yourself, when something is yours or comes from you or when it is not also, so in this way, be aware and let it go if appropriate. In recognition comes acceptance of what is, we only have this moment, the answers are not from here; however, you will find and access them. Remember that this is the moment that lasts.

Man and woman are made in the image and likeness, their own nature reveals it. Therefore, accepting nature as it is, is accepting human nature as a revelation. Acceptance is equilibrium and being the observer, you allow yourself to reach serenity, the indescribable, consciousness and beyond.

The acceptance of who you are, allows you to find your life purpose, integrating the being, on all levels, bodies, dimensions, realities and relativities in space-time. Acceptance is also the understanding, the consecration of the word as a principle of unity. Consecrate the enlightened word of love in you; the sacred word that originates from thought. Where brain coherence connect with the heart.

Forgiveness occurs when you understand under the principle of unity, that everything was as it had and had to be, that it could not be differently, regardless of how it was, the principle was executed, manifested and integrated even in what we perceive as chaos, conflict, illness, separation, etc. We do not grant forgiveness to anyone, it is as if we said that we forgive love; love is love, and all there is, is infinite love.

The expected moment has arrived, and the recognition and establishment of love in your heart they already are. Let go of everything that is prevalent and unnecessary, you no longer occupy it. Living the ecstasy of life, that is deserving. Living the ecstasy of what every act of love entails, that is deserving. Love is not suffering, but would cease to be in its main part and in its essential effect applied to the great masses.

The total count of our acts of life is and was, as it is, with nothing to add or take away from it, this is how it had to be in order to advance to the next step of our human evolution, from past times and from all realities. Everything has been so perfect as it has been and as it is. We are made for each other, we are not separate, we are one; the intrinsic separation between love and you is nothing.

It all comes down to love, light and yourself, in that triangular simplicity. That you only emit gratitude and arrive when you realize that you are aware of what has been done and what is already. Observe, thank, accept and continue; just seeing beyond, will allow you to be an observer of the manifestation of love in all its forms, the way in which everything converges towards the one, and the one with everything.

Recognize that the repetition of events in their multiple interpretations, places, and dimensions exist in all their forms in you. Therefore, you have created your own reality and only understanding it, you will stop judging, reproaching and blaming others for your own actions. Through the experience of others, we integrate; each one owns and has responsibility for his own actions; the whole is you. The manifestation of love in all its forms is to thank the noblest energy that can exist. Thank your day, your night, your feelings and your life. Make a chain of a thousand thanks.

The observer's acts

These acts are related to the brain and brain power. Neuroakashic® cellular fuels lead us to the integration of the actions of the observer towards the great observer. Allow yourself to observe the event, situation or circumstance and the way in which the principles of unity act and that those who transform themselves are us, at the moment when we allow ourselves and open ourselves to be and transform ourselves into the great observer.

The observer's acts are: the first act is to recognize and allow to observe yourself, observe your breathing. In the second act, it is allowing to recognize and observe yourself outside your field; the third act is to allow you to observe yourself from the great mountain as shown in figure 3. They are the cellular fuels that allow us to integrate these acts without judgment and expectations towards the 4th. act the great observer.

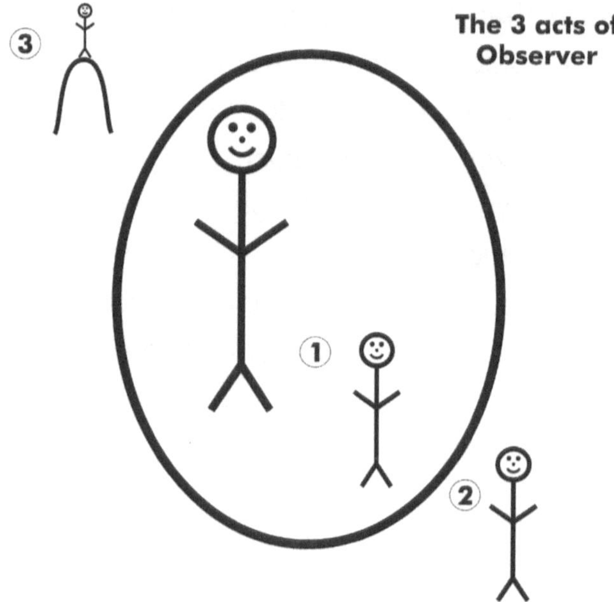

The objective is to stay as observers within the field, *I allow myself to be an observer inside or outside the field*; and convert ourselves from the observer to the great observer, which is to observe from something bigger. There will be certain situations that you are going to live or people that will come into your life, that will reflect you and will show and reveal how your n+1 field is, how your heart is and how you are from within. The observer realizes what is happening in the field and only maintains the observation without intervening.

The moment of the observer is already, stop carrying or feel that you carry something that apparently is not, observe and give yourself only for this instant this moment. It often happens that things are not as we wish them to be, note that no one has disappointed you, just note that something bigger is accommodating. Allowing you to see the light in you is the same light that is in the environment and allows them to see that light in you. Accept things as they are and let something bigger settle. If you are in a moment of decision, allow yourself to be only under the influence of love.

Realize, accept, understand and observe the world really as it is. Begins to observe through nonphysical eyes and begins to transform your perception and begin to evolve; evolution never stops, it is constantly advancing in evolution itself. The observer discovers himself and discovers why he is here, what he came to do and its interrelation with the inexhaustible source of love.

The observer, the world, the universe, the network systems and the great akashic® matrix, will teach the possibility of knowing that something else exists, which allow to connect with the infinite, without much effort to achieve it. The observer opens to connect with the source and with the real world to connect with divine energy; he gives himself up and flows, achieving a true divine experience.

The secret to connect is to give for yourself and then give

and integrate in expansion to the environment, working on the principles of unity, giving with your vehicle, foundation, engine and motive. What the observer requires, is projected in the network system; When the observer becomes the great observer, the level of consciousness is achieved, the hyper high Neuroakashic® potential, which is where co-creative and creative power, pleasure, balance, kindness and the principles of unity are activated.

CHAPTER 2

Neuroakashic®
Potential Balance

The great akashic® matrix

> "Like two drops of water, take the concepts
> into the void, let go and let loose."

> Ana Silvia Lara.

Have you ever wondered what the universe is and how it works? This book presents the other view of what the universe is, for us it is the great network system contained in the great akashic® matrix. It is approached from the transformative language, so I ask you to open your heart and mind to be able to integrate the corresponding process for you, where there is something bigger, called the great akashic® matrix which is to access the conductive and holographic super conductive computer towards or to the big universe. Welcome everyone to this great universe Neuroakashic®.

The great akashic® matrix (GAM) or akashic® for us, is a great machine that contains the DNA chains and integrates all the network systems, and these, in turn, contain the akashic® transformers and their interrelation with the n+1 fields, these are the sum of all the fields.

The GAM has other names such as: soul, high grace, essence, direct source; among others; it is a maximum divine intelligence, manifested and expanded, it is ineffable, unlimited and immeasurable, it is the mirror that opens and is born from the heart. It is the origin of everything and everything, the union of the heavenly with the earthly, is the bridge of transformation. It has different moments within the evolution process, since they have a magnificent degree of wisdom and it helps us evolve.

The functions of the GAM are: catalyst, conductive, encoder, amplifier, maximizer, replicator, transformer, generator, observer, mediator, actor, aligner, translator, high voltage capacitor, and usher. The GAM is and has been, has walked and has done it for centuries and thousands of years, finding itself, with its purest and original essence, with its other part to reach unicity.

He obeys the instinct of love, no matter his journey, he transcends his evolution ladder, he never stops, his learning which is love, never ends since everything is. The GAM cannot transgress, remove, eliminate the history that it keeps, rather of understanding, wisdom of light and integrating the whole and achieving unicity.

From the encounter with its origin, to space-time, in all its existence. To encounter with her most sacred, purest, which is her own light. The configuration or networks-configuration is balanced, to the encounter with love. Unifying the consciousness of the whole. Consciousness is light, because in the purity of love is light.

In Figure 4, the great akashic® matrix is shown:

Great Akashic® Matrix

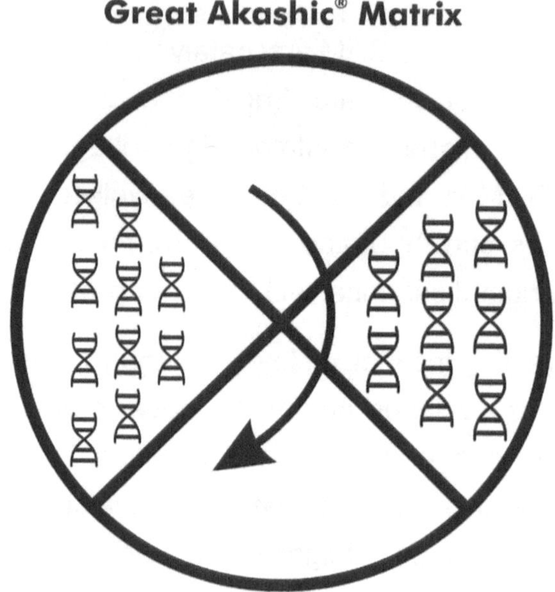

In Figure 5, the great akashic® matrix is seen as the set of all network systems, in all lines and cycles of space-time, where the user's field is interrelated. The connection to the great akashic® matrix works in 3 ways: 1) the light connects to and from the helm (great akashic® matrix); 2) from the controller or control panel *expandia* irrigates towards the heart, as we will see later on; 3) the akashic® transformer connects with the spinal cord and the endocrine system, the glands: pituitary, pineal, thymus, thyroid and parathyroid.

Great Akashic® Matrix

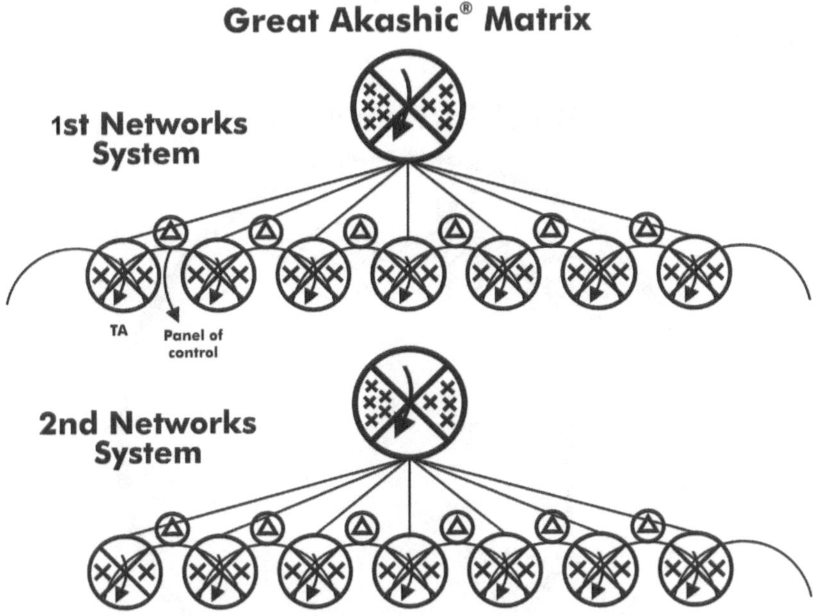

The akashic® transformer shown in figure 6, is a machine that contains all the interdimensional bridges of DNA, (DNA and RNA chains) is the storage of light of all times and realities. These transformers are part of the great Neuroakashic® network system, which integrates all the respective network systems and corresponding to the great akashic® matrix.

This akashic® transformer is another machine contained in network systems in the great akashic® matrix and it works in two ways or in two paths, since the transmitter box connects to the central nervous system to the switches and connectors at their maximum power in two ways: The first way: connects with the central nervous system, particularly the brain and in the upper part of the brain, and covers the connected right and left cerebral hemispheres and reaches the coccyx. The second way: it is located in the brain stem and communicates with the spinal cord and peripheral nerves, connects with the heart as shown in figure 6.

Akashic® Transformer

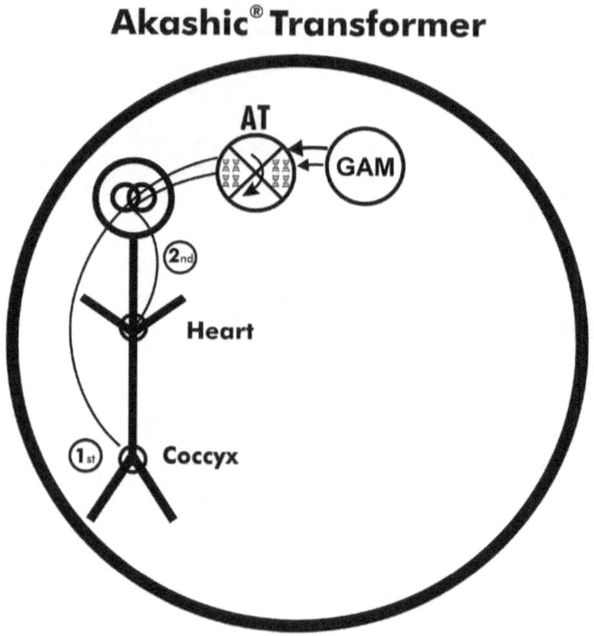

Authors have named the great akashic® matrix as: Ermano Paoelli as a unified field of information, for Pribram the holographic universe, for Gregg Braden it is called the divine matrix. For Bohm, it becomes a kind of great universal mind, a holographic mind or program, in which the past, present and future coexist simultaneously. For Nikola Tesla, it is the sun, the great source of light, with a rotating electromagnetic field as a great inexhaustible source of energy.

For Gregg Braden, his understanding of Planck's matrix, describing it as a form of energy that is everywhere; the existence of this field implies three principles: all things exist within the divine matrix, they are connected, it must have an effect and an influence on all the parts. This for us, the replicity and synchronicity effect of the n+1 fields.

Lattice for Jacobo Grinberg, according to the sintergic theory, is a structure, hyper complex network or energy matrix with levels of micro and macro particles; therefore, the interaction with the sintergic bands, are for us the network systems. The lattice is for us the great akashic® matrix, and it is interrelated with Neuroakashic® because it can explain the functionality, the degrees, the operability of the n+1 fields in network systems.

Thus, the lattice arises from the result of the interaction between the neural field and the lattice of space-time; the evidence about the superconducting character comes from the Aspect experiment (1982), which is based on the Einstein-Rosen-Podolsky paradox. For Jacobo Grinberg lattice, it is superconducting and holographic and if the brain is a replica of the universe or lattice, the brain is also holographic and superconducting. (Grinberg, 1988, pg. 46, 48).

How is the brain's superconducting and holographic capacity measured as a function of mother earth? Through the relation with the crystals as we will see later.

Thus, the great akashic® matrix is the process of connection or similarity of the system, it is a networked computer, which manifests itself as the great replica to the brain. Therefore, the brain is in replication and in connection with the universe, it has a relation to the central crystal of mother earth.

The brain is in relation to the n+1 fields (sum of all fields) of mother earth, Gaia and the central crystal of mother earth and hence its connection to the cerebral hemispheres, heart, intestines, coccyx and again central crystal from mother earth, this is the flow of life. So, the great akashic® matrix is superconducting and holographic as the brain is, since the brain is the replica of the universe and this universe is the great akashic® matrix and the network systems as a whole as shown in the figure 7.

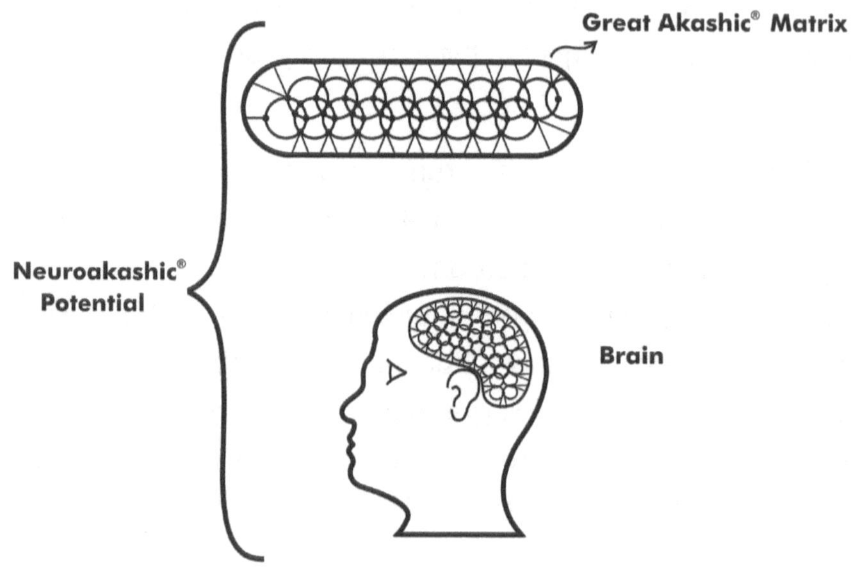

Evolution of the brain to Neuroakashic®

The brain is the great central machine, it is the great computer that is made up of a great network of neurons; it is the control center of the entire central nervous system, it is like the power station, the great super computer and mainframe. Thus, the great human brain with all its complexity and its neural network system, is the great machine in replication of the great akashic® matrix. Pibram and Ramírez mention that the human brain is a multiprogrammer and multiprocessor system (Pibram and Ramirez, 1980, pg. 16)

For Hamer in the summary of the new medicine, he mentioned that the brain is the central supercomputer, it is the encoder of the organs and the control panel of the cells, in addition there is a correlation between the triad: psyche, organ and focus (short circuit) the breakdown of the electrophysiological field in the brain and where Neuroakashic® works at the level of the user's n+1 field, balancing network systems from brain, heart, intestines, coccyx, among other.

In theory, MacLean's triune brain in 1978 mentions that the first reptilian brain or cerebellum is characterized and based on instincts; the second limbic or emotional brain is one that is based on emotions; the third brain, neocortex or cerebral cortex, which are the left and right hemisphere.

Starting from this, there is the bridge (as seen in figure 7), which represents the lessons, learnings, environments, circumstances, tools, that lead us to the awakening and expansion of consciousness; it leads us to something greater, to realize without intervening, to judge, to compare, to analyze or to separate, it is to give way to the integrating, renewing and transforming process.

It takes us to the next link in the evolution of humanity, in the neural brain evolution, we call it Neuroakashic®, which comes from neuro in neuron as potential action and akashic® or great akashic® matrix is the great machine that contains the neural networks systems and great network systems. We then call the Neuroakashic® potential, the balance of the neural network systems between the brain, heart and intestines; there are levels or degrees of brain potential or Neuroakashic® potential, also called level of consciousness, the harmonic state or coherence.

Akashic Activator® Unlimited Light®, is a cellular fuel, which balances both the cerebral hemispheres, the creative and emotional right and the logical and rational left. Balancing the cerebral hemispheres, in the harmonic or coherent state, in order to manifest balance, peace, love, expansion, compassion, empathy and harmony.

For Fuster, the prefrontal cortex is the memory of the future. In addition, the cortex develops educational, scientific, artistic, legislative, sports initiatives, etc. (Fuster, 2015 pg. 52, 73). This, is proper to achieve the balance of the brain in hyper high Neuroakashic® potential, since it manages to enable, develop, integrate and enhance high capacities or superior capacities, such as we will see later.

The Evolution Neuroakashic®

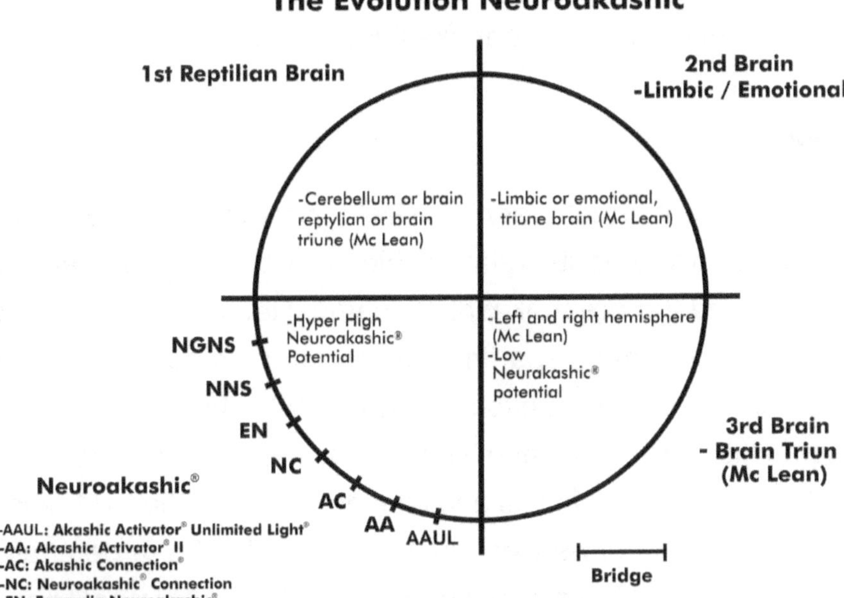

Pineal gland

The pineal gland is connected to and receives signals from akashic® transformers in network systems that function as emitters and transducers; This signal and holographic property comes from the great akashic® matrix, which connects to transformers and interrelated network systems. The pineal gland is also connected to the control or information panel called *expandia*, from the network systems that make up the great akashic® matrix to the pineal gland.

Subsequently, to the cerebral hemispheres, to the heart, intestines, coccyx and to the central crystal of mother earth, this last one, are the cerebral hemispheres, to fulfill the vital flow of life. Therefore, the pineal gland plays an important role in the Neuroakashic® process since it is the connection or the link to connect to the great akashic® matrix.

DNA

The great machinery of DNA, contained in akashic® transformers, and its relationship with the central nervous system and the great akashic® matrix. Neuroakashic® works from the genome, repairing the chromosomes and can be corrected from the mitochondrial DNA chains and in its metabolism. The DNA and RNA chains are related to the user's n+1 field (sum of all fields) and in relation to the other n+1 fields, with the effects of network systems. That is, the large chains of DNA and RNA are contained in the akashic® transformers and these within the network systems and this last ones in the great akashic® matrix.

We have observed both in the user, as the observer or practitioner of Neuroakashic® training, as well as the way in which they integrate superior capacities or high capacities, born talents. Therefore, in addition, the impact of sharing Neuroakashic® is *n* times more in n+1 fields, that is, the impact it has on great network systems is immeasurable.

DNA and Central Crystal
of Mother Earth
(Brain hemispheres)

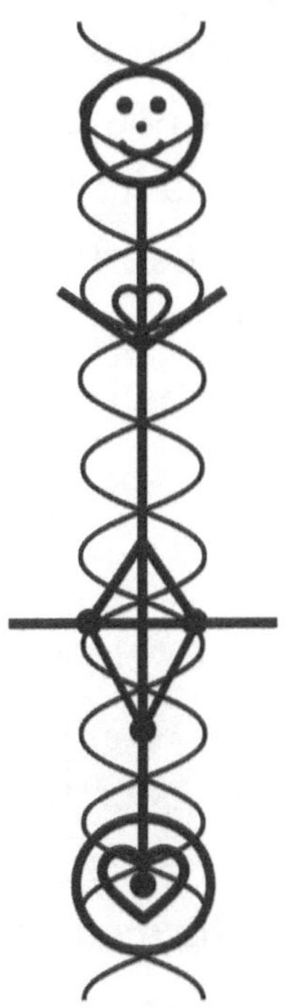

The central crystal of mother earth
(cerebral hemispheres)

It is related and closely linked to brain (neuronal) activity. In other words, Neuroakashic® promotes and activates brain activity and the neuronal synapse and, as a whole, the neural network system and the central nervous system. The central crystal of the mother earth, are the cerebral hemispheres that are balanced and allow to observe and integrate other realities. Through the pituitary gland, the evolutionary, rapid and immediate flows.

The greater the anchorage, the greater the evolution of everything, what is and exists is infinite, without a beginning or end; everything expands and amplifies at incredible speeds. Everything in nothing, nothing in everything. During Neuroakashic® sessions, it has been observed how energy moves from top to bottom and from bottom to top, that is, from the cerebral hemispheres, heart, intestines, coccyx, central crystal of mother earth and vice versa, as through photonic light it moves energy or information to networks in space-time.

Maternal womb

This refers to an intrinsic relationship between the neural network systems and the coccyx, intestines, uterus, belly and womb. The womb and the coccyx are the accumulators of energy; This explains the relationship and existence of the akashic® transformer. It is the mother's womb, the place where this accumulator of feminine energy is found and which is linked to the heart and to everything.

With the use of energy, it can reduce network systems and the corresponding electricity voltages. Therefore, Neuroakashic® fuels help to adjust, balance, equilibrate the belly, intestines, heart and cerebral hemispheres connected to the great network system.

Central Nervous System

The central nervous system in a harmonic state, connected to akashic® transformers, which integrate network systems and are in motion all the time. Scientists Pribram and Ramírez mention that brain physiologists have shown that the nervous system is a frequency analyzer, in the manner of a holographic pattern (Pribram and Ramirez, 1980, pg.107).

For us, the central nervous system is the one that receives the signals from the akashic® transformers connected to the network system and the great akashic® matrix, and from there it sends signals to the rest of the organism, to the heart, intestines, coccyx, central crystal from mother earth (refers to the cerebral hemispheres). That is, the central nervous system is connected to the central crystal of mother earth, back and forth to the cerebral hemispheres.

This system is the replicator and transformer, which has an intrinsic relationship with the control panel, we call it expandia and it's also called information panel connected to great network systems. The central nervous system is the spearhead for the major anchorage and the connection to the great akashic® matrix, with our mother earth planet Gaia and with ourselves.

Likewise, this is the watershed, to achieve the balance of the Neuroakashic® potential, in which the alterations and imbalance of the central nervous system, rootlessness and greater anchorage are integrated. Grinberg mentioned that the nervous system acts as the antenna of consciousness and that it also detects the coherence changes of the lattice, manifesting them before our perception of sensations of approaching or distancing, with respect to objects or the perception of speed and acceleration. (Grinberg, 1991, pg. 18)

Cases of students who presented the capacity or perception of acceleration and of unfolding events, objects, circumstances and of integrating other realities that are happening at the same time were manifested; this is explained through changes in the high or hiper high levels of coherence or Neuroakashic® potential.

It has been observed, as adjustments are made in various disorders and pathologies related to the central nervous system, that some degenerative, neurological, psychological, and psychiatric diseases may develop due to affectations in the nervous system. Neuroakashic® activates and regenerates the central nervous system, works the neurogenesis process, with the aim of generating new additional nerve cells, as well as balancing alterations in neuronal and psychiatric migration.

Neuroplasticity

Neuroplasticity is the potential of the nervous system to mold itself and form new nerve connections. It is also the ability of cells and neurons to adapt and to transform to change. For Joe Dispenza, neuroplasticity is the ability to reconnect and create new neural circuits, it is the ability to be neuroplastic, equivalent to the ability to change our minds. (Dispenza, 2008, pg. 10)

Furthermore, it can redesign and reconfigure neural network systems, adapting to changes and movement of networks. The increase in neuroplasticity is favorable in relation to the use of Neuroakashic® fuels, it manages to maintain and balance and increase neuronal synaptic plasticity, which is the connection and communication of neurons; allowing balance in oxidative stress, maintaining and promoting neuronal regeneration and the birth of new neurons (neurogenesis).

Through brain neuroplasticity, being observers from the great observer, stay under the principles of unity, to develop and potentiate your superior capacities, developing and increasing brain potential. Likewise, improve the performance of the brain, knowing yourself and enhancing your gifts, abilities, and other potentials to improve your quality of life in balance, fulfillment.

On the other hand, Neuroakashic® balances brain neuroplasticity together with plasticity and genome stability, in order to achieve the genomic sequence. Akashic Activator® Unlimited Light®, works from the cell membrane, cellular communication and particularly the neural, as well as being a cell rejuvenator and preventing aging.

Neurons

Neurons, are the energy units that are the transmitters of information in great neural network systems, are the great cellular machinery of the central nervous system. For Fuster, a neuron is an electrically excitable cell in the central nervous system that processes and transmits information using electrical and chemical signals. (Fuster, 2015, pg. 359)

Therefore, neurons, are connected and interconnected in network systems, there are billions of neurons in the human brain, they are a type of cell that represents the structural and functional unit of the central nervous system. Neurons transmit information in network systems, that is, they act as detoxifiers, cleaners, integrators and adjusters of the environment in the network system, bringing information to the organs and systems of the body, forming and creating new cells in unison.

The key is to keep neurons alive, in balance with neuronal communication, keep the neuronal system in motion, stable neurons, since the purpose is the genesis, and reestablish the neurons that die, to avoid neuronal death, which It causes due to various factors such as oxidative stress, diet, habits, belief systems, among others. And thus achieve an optimal state of health in users.

The cell is the transmitter and vehicle of light, it is the vehicle and mechanism of the network system, from the mitochondrial cell. Another type of cells, are glial cells, which have a great influence encoding through light, here the neurons, the brain and their processing or system of neural networks are interconnected.

Neurons carry out processes of brain integration, which occurs from neural systems and circuits and photonic light, triggering the process of balancing the Neuroakashic® potential, that great network of divine particles that make up the universe, that make up the n+1 fields, it has its holographic property with pure and coherent laser light.

Neuroakashic®, from the Akashic Activator® Unlimited Light® process, works from the nucleus and cell membrane. The biohematic cellular catalyst aims to purify blood cells, since there is information in it, the same information that travels through signals from the central nervous system and neurons.

Neurotransmitters

Neuroakashic® balances neurotransmitters, since a decrease or rise in their level can cause some psychological, psychiatric and neurological disorders, high levels of depression and high levels of violence. A greater balance of brain power or Neuroakashic® potential, the process and principle of giving is balanced and integrated, the greater connection to mother earth, the greater level of balance in levels of rootlessness and greater anchorage.

Neurotransmitters are related to the cerebral hemispheres and their relationship to neural network systems and levels of rootlessness and major anchorage. For Fuster, the neurotransmitter is an endogenous chemical, which transmits information from one neuron to another through its membranes. (Fuster, 2015, pg. 359).

The purpose is to balance neurotransmitters such as oxytocin considered the love hormone. Recalling that the greater the balance of the neurotransmitters, the greater the creative power; if there is a decrease in neurotransmitters, therefore, it decreases. In conclusion, the more light there is in the neurotransmitters that are produced, the greater the light of expansion and growth.

Immune system

It is vitally important to strengthen the immune system and its relationship to neural network systems, great network systems, and how the glands, including the thymus gland, are related to the development of consciousness, as it is the round-trip transmitter, connected to network systems; one of its functions is to purify and tighten its connection with neural network systems.

Thus, it is the immune system it is the motor in the neural network system, it is also itself a network system, so, through Neuroakashic®, it strengthens the immune system and mitigates oxidative stress, physical stress, mental stress, emotional stress, of the most common diseases today, can cause neuronal death and other pathologies.

It was observed that cancer users who received sessions of Neuroakashic® alternated with their medical treatment, reported decreased effects on radiation or chemotherapy. Today, you are receiving your sessions continuously and balancing your level of brain power or Neuroakashic® potential, to feel well-being, balanced, consistent every day. So you have to observe the cells and how the cycles are adjusting and accommodating.

Immune System

Brain waves

> If you want to discover the secrets
> of the universe, think in terms of
> energy, frequency and vibration.
>
> Nikola Tesla

Brain waves are the electrical activity produced by the brain, and the types of brain waves are: Delta, Theta, Alpha, Beta, and Gamma. Neuroakashic® works on gamma waves, they are the fuel for our neurons, there is a close relationship between neural effects, waves and neural networks. From the spinal column and root chakra, to the heart. The n+1 fields (as the sum of all the fields) are prepared in advance to be observed in these processes.

The benefits of gamma waves are: memory, concentration, super-developed intuition, high-level cognitive state, compassion, feeling of happiness, remote vision, development of advanced meditative states, and amplification of neural signaling and perception of other realities. The secret is to maintain the gamma waves, so that the corresponding adjustments are made at the level of neural network systems.

It can be seen that Neuroakashic® induces brain waves to change their frequency to gamma waves. Scientists Sciotto and Niripil mention that these are high frequency waves, from 40 hertz or more; in addition to being brain waves, they are the set of electrical signals that our neurons emit.

There is a relationship between brain waves and the heart, since the process of balancing the Neuroakashic® potential level and brain coherence is related to the heart and the relationship to the n+1 field, Gaia, the relationship to the n+1 field, mother earth and in relation to ourselves. We can say then, that there is a close relationship of brain waves, the n+1 fields and the magnetic field of mother earth. What allows us to observe today the universe as it is, or as it has been.

Neuroakashic®, works on gamma waves, in person or remotely. In online mode, it has been observed that the signal expands and amplifies in network systems, from the capacity of the great observer. While our thoughts, emotions and feelings are related to brain waves, through Neuroakashic®, we can balance ourselves through these waves, so that our thoughts are balanced and in a harmonic state.

Mind

> The field is the only ruling entity
> of the particle, the mind is the
> only ruling entity of the body.
>
> Einstein

When harmonic balance is achieved, thought and emotion are one, in unity with the heart and brain. What the mind has perceived as resistance as limitation only exists in the separation, observe how it integrates into you. Observe how the principles of unity are integrated, the principle of non-separation, about time, love, etc. The brain is the great source of inspiration.

Observe the mind and its relationship with the observer, is integrated into the study of neuroakashic® network systems.

The mind creates the thoughts and these thoughts are the reality, the mental state can be altered by one or more elements or components of the n+1 fields in the network systems. The mind is also part of these n+1 fields of the environment, the interrelation of the n+1 fields are with other n+1 fields, and other respective and corresponding network systems, forming unity. Thought is light and light is thought. Light is projected into images and connected to thought.

Fields

The field comes from the earth, from interaction with nature, with animals, with the elements, and from there arises the n+1 field, the union of all fields, without distinction or separation. For us, the n+1 field is the way to call the sum of all the fields, all the signals in the field are an opportunity.

Bruce Lipton mentions that in quantum physics and in today's world, spirit and field are the same. Lynne Mctaggart, in her work "The Field", the structure of DNA has a surrounding field, known as an electromagnetic field, in which one field versus another field generates an interference field.

Here, it coincides with Nikola Tesla's resonance theory, in which one field is affected by the other field. And this also coincides with our theory of n+1 fields, in network systems. Jacobo Grinberg calls it the neural field is the activity of a living brain that results from the interactions of the neural elements that form it.

Theory of the n+1 field

For the n+1 field to exist, before there was unity, subatomic particles and atoms, particles of photons, neutrons, protons, etc. All this set acting in a holographic way impacting the n+1 fields, this field is the sum of all the fields, which generally encompasses the field of the user, the place, state, country, planet, universe, mother earth, Gaia. This theory is the one we are currently sharing, the one that indicates our acts and actions, having repercussions in the n+1 field, n times, that is, it has a great influence on the alternate fields.

If there is a great influence from the field to the observer and from the observer to the n+1 field, there will be an effect in both and in the n+1 field, and if it is visualized, a model and a formula of access to networks and consciousness of unity. Three elements will be dealt with in the field: 1) level of consciousness or Neuroakashic® potential, 2) the acts of the great observer, 3) anchoring the word in the field.

It is not only necessary to take into account the past, but also the replicity of the n+1 fields and retake the fields that are in network connection. Observe the synchronicity and replicity of events or circumstances in field n+1. It begins to anchor through the word, in the n+1 fields, through the overall and inclusive transforming language, the one that makes up the n+1 fields and the great network system.

Thus, the integrating principles of the energy of giving, of money, of love, of cycles and time lines are already there. Everything that is issued verbally or written to this field is housed there; therefore, our work is to observe how the process of adjustment of accommodation and solution is carried out in the respective and corresponding network system. What we do today will impact tomorrow, or future and future generations. So, the expansive conscious process of love begins today.

The n+1 field shows some feelings that are adjusting, such as adjusting love and work relationships. Be observant and integrate the relationship over time. The networking movement started in advance, even before reading this book, there was a preparation for everyone, to be in the n+1 field Neuroakashic®, and observing this transformative process in you.

The interaction of the n+1 fields are fields in constant expansion with other fields and from these emerge and create alterations in the networks. We have observed that it is not enough to balance the neurotransmitters, is something else happening?, the transformation to the harmonic state, promotes the equable energy flow of the neurotransmitters for the relationship or interrelation with the gamma waves and achieve being in balance, observing from the great observer in the n+1 fields.

Interrelation of the n+1 field

The field, the situations and the day-to-day experiences are affected by the n+1 fields, what manifests itself is a reflection of ourselves, so we ourselves are the n+1 fields, the sound waves, the energy, the rays of light, frequency, vibration that is what connects and is reflected in the network systems and the great akashic® matrix, how from a cell and neuron they are connecting to the network systems.

We are the fusion of sound waves with the whole, and not a separation, we are the integration of the whole, from the micro and macro level, connected to the great universe Neuroakashic®. From cells and neurons, it made its amplitude in all its splendor, from the brain level you are a thought, therefore a thought at a micro or macro level, can expand the network systems and you can vibrate that thought in the network system and managing to be perceived by users and the environment.

We are the set of cells, neurons, thoughts, all this interconnected; we are that wave of energy that is reflected in the n+1 field, we are ourselves. For this effect, what is reflected in the n+1 field is the result of ourselves, we are thoughts connected from Neuroakashic® balance, in order to develop and enhance our gifts, talents, superior abilities and skills to connect and integrate to network systems, and the n+1 fields.

Therefore, as you work with Neuroakashic®, the more connected you are to your own reality, the more connected you are to all the implications of the n+1 fields, due to their importance in understanding and discerning what is happening right there. It is important to highlight the openness to understanding how fields work in this theory of n+1 fields.

Neuroakashic® can help you connect with yourself and with the whole, making the appropriate structural adjustments, to connect through light and all network systems. Be the observer of everything that happens day by day with the n+1 fields, observe the interrelation and interpretation of the n+1 fields, without intervention and from the harmonic, fair and impeccable state.

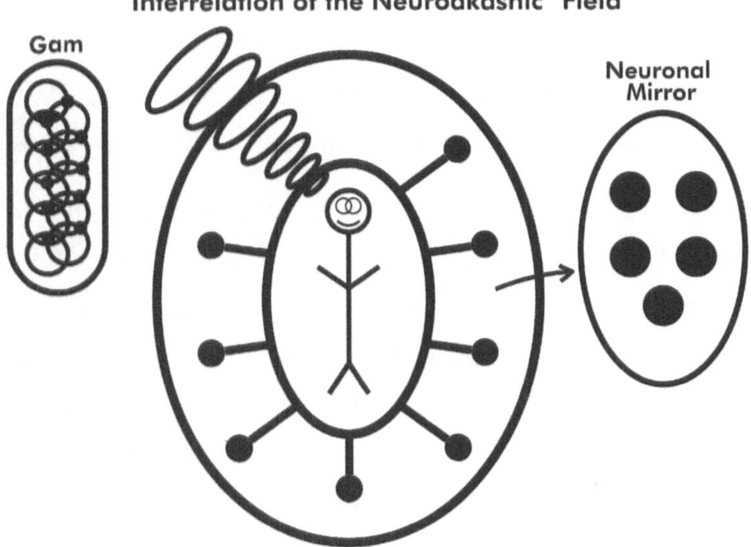

The transformation of the n+1 fields

Our field is intertwined from the great akashic® matrix and the DNA of the first man and the first woman. We are living a reality in multiple realities, living a moment that we have lived and repeated hundreds or thousands of times in the n+1 fields of network systems; we have repeated the same scene, the same event, n times in the history of humanity, in the various lines, cycles of time and realities. Our origin is love. Stop preventing things from happening, give yourself to the field and it transforms everything.

Love itself will unite us again, even if centuries or eternities pass, what corresponds to each one arrives in the coherent, progressive, transforming and integrative evolutionary process. It is suggested that observing what we cannot change and observing the golden rule is what corresponds, corresponds what is. Observe, accept, thank and continue; it is important to maintain ourselves from the act of the observer, of what happens within the n+1 field and outside it, since it is not the same to be within it, as outside observing and even more so from the great observer.

This is where the importance of becoming and transforming in the great observer lies. Without the act of the observer, you will be able to hook yourself with what you manifest in the field, from that family, the house, the place, the city, the state, the country or the planet. For example, any feeling corresponds to the n+1 field or to the environment itself, in all the cycles and lines of space-time, just be observant.

Synchronicity and holographic replicity in n+1 fields

All realities are embodied in each other. The fields follow a synchronicity in perfect symbiotic relationship that is formed in the network system. When you help connect someone else, we are connected *to something bigger,* in all directions. When you are the observer, you realize that you are connected to something bigger. The self is integrated and unified, to the whole, from your inner child, from your life story, until today.

An n+1 field can be replicated to another, that is, what manifests in one field is replicated in another, since they can be transferred or synchronized with others and in other realities of space-time. An n+1 field has a reflection that is its own matrix or nucleus, within n fields referred to each other. Everything is a tiny infinite part of everything.

The situation, event or circumstance of what happens in the n+1 field, resonates with the user somewhere in himself and transform the dysfunctionalities in the corresponding network systems. Being the observer, you can observe those situations, events, circumstances that correspond to the corresponding field. So it is suggested to remain an observer and observe the field.

An n+1 field can be replicated earlier, that is, how the effect manifests in the field and then the cause, and this is replicated *n* times in other alternate fields. So, you can know what is going to happen, due to this movement in the network systems. A situation, event, circumstance can be replicated in several other fields, but even love is running on the corresponding network system.

Another term worth highlighting is *holographic replication in the n+1 field*. It can be described as an effect, event or circumstance, it is replicated *n* more times in *n* different fields.

Holographic Replicity in the N + 1 field

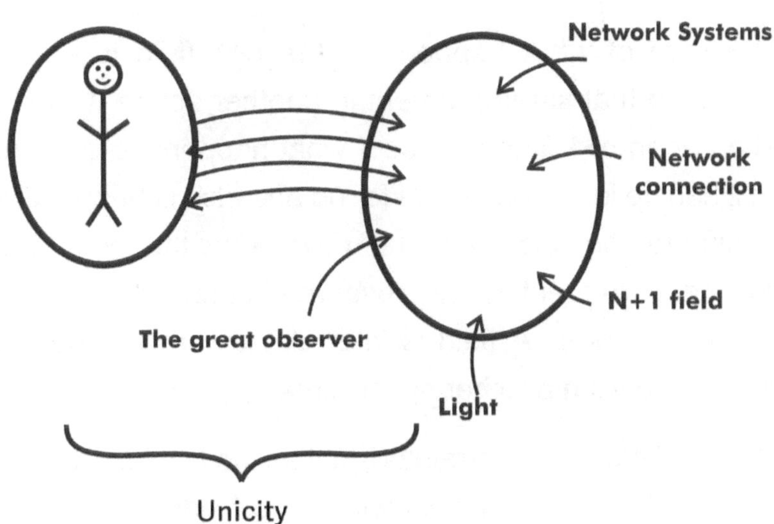

There is no probability, when there is certainty, this last means that the succession of various elements or components within the field can never be. There will always be alteration or modification. The question is, how and what can be altered in the field? And who issues the first or last message? The answer to this is that the first message is not the same as the last. So, there is alteration from the message and who sends it also in the network systems.

In other words, the message will never be the same since there is involvement, movement and interrelation of various $n+1$ fields in the great network system. It is also possible to predict the behavior of the $n+1$ field over and over again. The photonic light is the one that emanates from the $n+1$ field, back and forth. The same field will give you the answers of what you require or are required through the signals in the $n+1$ fields.

Symbiotic relationship of the $n+1$ field

The sum of what happens in the $n+1$ field is equal to everything in that same moment in another space. When the vibration of an $n+1$ field is raised, what happens to each user within it can be identified. What for no one else is happening, is happening for the field itself. The movements that occur within the $n+1$ field are created and observed in network connection in network systems. A field is interrelated with another field, even if it were from another space-time.

The $n+1$ fields are interrelated, just as the last field is related to the first, that is, the events within the fields are related to each other, on the same line or time cycles. The observer has the ability to observe and interrelate the networks in the fields. The anchorage in the field, is the word, when you are an observer, and the acts of the observer are performed, it is observed how what is directed or perceived in the field is linked to something larger such as the n+1 field.

The sum of what happens in the n+1 field, is equal to the whole of that same moment in another space, in an n+1 field you can identify and observe what happens to each user within it; what no one else can see with the physical eyes or in a tangible way, is already happening for the field itself.

The movements that occur within the n+1 field are created and observed in the network connection of network systems. There are signals that manifest the n+1 field in advance, likewise the event in a synchronicity effect, can occur and manifest what the user experiences as interference from the outside.

Practical case

It was done through a computer, it was observed that this device connects the image from and coming from the brain, the idea or thought is emitted by the user, it is sent in an ascending line of the brain and it is projected on the cell phone, we call this holographic brain, when the word is emitted, a neuronal synapse is sent and made with the neural networks. There is an interrelation of the n+1 fields, since the ability to see or perceive through non-physical eyes, remote vision, is manifested and reflected in the n+1 field. The hologram is projected onto the field and the interrelation of these fields is given.

An exercise was performed with two people who have taken the Neuroakashic® training, each student using a computer, and the results were: in the first exercise, a word was chosen and this was chosen by student A), who named *love*, (comments that he visualized on a website, the word longing). Student B) commented that she found the phrase: *connect more with love.*

In the 2nd. exercise, the word "nature" was chosen, which was chosen by student B); the first student A) reports that she perceived the image of nature and longing on the same website. While student B) reports having found the image of the first exercise, finding love and in the second image nature, which she found on another page that she browsed.

In the 3rd. exercise, the word "eyes" was chosen, this last word was chosen by student A), who reveals that this image was observed from above the image of longing. Student B) reports having found the eye image. In the case of student A), and manifested the holographic image and remote viewing of this exercise. In the case of student B), she could have influenced her belief system to slow down and find the image on the website, receiving a phrase instead of an image. Later, she found the image in the second exercise.

The brains of these two students were observed to be networked, interconnected in direct communication. It was also observed that the n+1 field of the word or image was directly related to the students, and in general in the n+1 field; both were related to the holographic images found.

That is, their brains were directly connected to the great akashic® matrix, The neural mirror of one student was reflected in the n+1 field of the other student and vice versa, both shared the neural flow. Another conclusion that was observed is that the brain projects to the cell phone or computer what is in its neural networks connected to something larger.

We conclude that the student or user has the control or influence of the processor or device to project any thought in the neural mirror. There can also be an influence of the environment of the n+1 field on the user, since an influence can be achieved from the user's and environment's thinking.

So, if the fields in general can be altered or manipulated in any way, it is because people connect with their emotions, thoughts and feelings and that can influence or be influenced by the test. That influence of the environment is what can move networks; it is suggested to work with Neuroakashic®, and the principles of unity, to be able to act as the observer, from the great observer.

It is suggested, to change proxy variable instead of computer or cell phone, we could take some object that would act as a mirror. Since what manifests in the field is holography, which is the light transformed into an image and that transmits what is in the field. It is important to observe the influence and impact of the n+1 fields on brain and neuronal activity, and the impact of the environment can influence the n+1 fields.

It is suggested to change the scenario and not to have contact with the users before carrying out the test. Identify the neural mirror and the relationship between the IQ and its relationship to the n+1 field. The impact of these tests and all our actions have a very significant impact today and tomorrow in the n+1 fields, as well as the impact of the Neuroakashic® potential on networks.

Another test was performed with a student who has not taken the Neuroakashic® training, in which, the student within the same field n+1, observed the influence of the observer within that same field, the exercises that were performed were not successful as the example above.

Finally, the exercise was carried out with the observer outside the field and from the great observer, as a result, the student was able to complete his exercises, resulting in the identification of the images on the internet pages, with the corresponding holograms, but without developing or manifest superior ability skills like expanded remote viewing and others.

Symbiotic Relationship of the N + 1 field

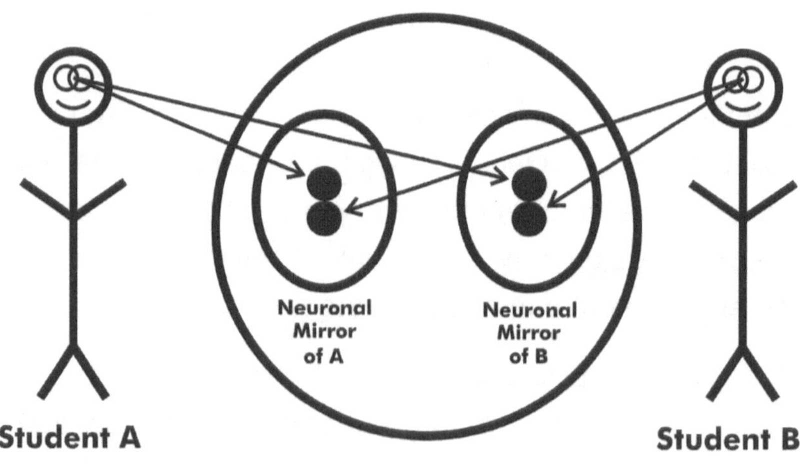

Divine actors

What a user experiences is not the effect or responsibility of others, he lives the result of how his heart is, how his relationship with himself is, in a mirror effect reflected in the n+1 field. In other words, what manifests in the n+1 field in your daily life is the result of the events, trajectory and environment manifested in the n+1 field, achieving a replica effect with the collective n+1 field.

Therefore, it is important that the observing being can discern, be within the field and outside it; and from the great observer integrate the influence of the n+1 fields of the collective consciousness. Learn to observe without judging, without indicting, without justifying, without manipulating, without controlling, without forcing, without expecting something or generating expectation, etc. The experiences with the divine actors who act, teach and reveal that we are already the great observer, that we are part of the whole of unity.

To understand the divine actors is to understand the environment itself, since it allows us to observe the way in which we are integrating ourselves with the great observer. Notice that some things belong to other related fields, even other networks from the great observer.

Motivated Field of action n+1

Great Akashic® Motivated Action Field

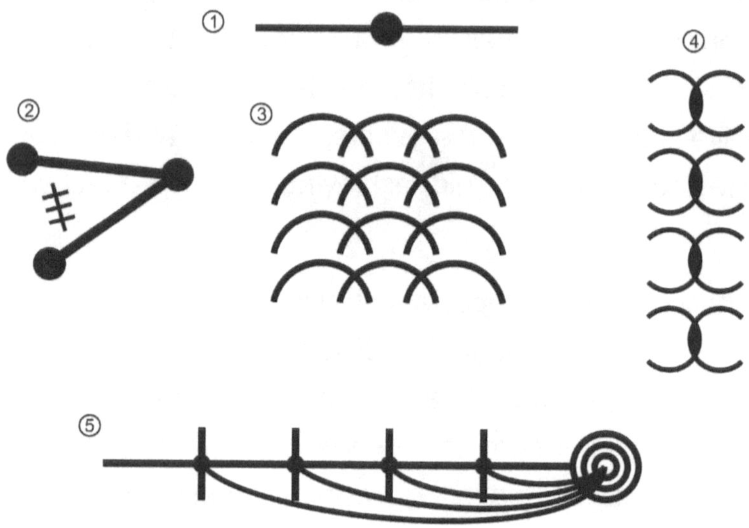

This field reflects love, the response of the field is already. Observe how it is done as follows:

1) It is identified within the n+1 field with the other elements

2) Permission is granted and connected to the great network system

3) Opening of the fields

4) Recognition, contact and approach of other components in the field

5) Interrelation with the elements and components that make up the field (from eye contact, verbal, mental, physical contact)

6) Confirmation of the elements and components to connect and integrate to the great main or direct source great akashic® matrix (GAM)

7) Confirmation and interrelation at the same time and integration to the whole. A movement of the network is made to find and stop at a point of balance.

8) It connects in a direct way to the great central network system, specifically to a network system and confirms the "positive or accredited" act of the past (of another moment or time).

9) It brings back the network system to the present moment, visually, audibly, odor, etc.

10) Observe the connection to other alternative network systems.

11) Connection, repetition, validation, corroboration to other network systems; an event traced from before is observed in the timeline and that forms a grouping and integrates.

All events on that same line and time cycles, - with respect to the elements, - were brought to the components in those network systems. Recognizing every event in the past, its elements and components. Each element and component are integrated in the recognition of the n+1 field, forming a large n+1 motivated field of action.

Neuroakashic® Potential (Level or degree of Consciousness)

The levels of consciousness are for us the Neuroakashic® potential, in which the level of the Neuroakashic® potential coexists, low, medium high, high and hyper level of consciousness. Jacobo Grinberg in his sintergic theory, talks about the brain with high neurosintergic and greater coherence and the low neurosintergic, less coherence; for us this is the high and low Neuroakashic® potential.

This latter is characterized by its structure, reason, judgment, expectations, conditioning, attachments, user intervention to control, manipulate, force, in addition to the belief system and the use of reason to explain and justify. For example, self-sacrifice, self-deception, self-sabotage, self-destruction that begins from your cells and from thought itself.

These degrees or levels of consciousness are also called harmonic state, coherence, brain power or Neuroakashic® potential, intrinsically related with the observer's acts. It exists a relationship between levels of consciousness, brain power, harmonic state, the actions of the Observer, the Tri-Une brain and the Neuroakashic® potential, as shown in the graph, figure 15:

Levels or degrees of consciousness			
Low Neuroakashic® potential (LNP)	Medium high Neuroakashic® potential (MHNP)	High Neuroakashic® potential (HNP)	Hyper high Neuroakashic® potential (HHNP) or Neuroakashic® potential equilibrium (NPE)
Low brain power (LBP)	Medium high brain power (MHBP)	High brain power (HBP)	Hyper high brain power (HHBP) or super high (SHBP)
Low level of consciousness (LLC)	Medium high level of consciousness (MHLC)	High level of consciousness (HLC)	Super or supra level of consciousness (SLC) or unity consciousness (UC)
Low coherence (LC)	Medium high coherence (MHC)	High coherence (HC)	Super high coherence (SHC) or hyper high (HHC)
Low harmonic state (LHS)	Medium high harmonic state (MHHS)	High harmonic state (HHS)	Super high or hyper high harmonic state (SHHS) (HHHS)
1st. Brain (Triune brain)	2nd. Brain (Triune brain)	3rd. Brain (Triune brain)	4th. Brain - heart (4BH)
1st. Act of the Observador (1AO)	2nd. Act of the Observer (2AO)	3rd. Act of the Observer (3AO)	4th. The Great Observer (4TGO)
Rootlessness level (RL) and hyper-high anchorage level (HHAL) from 11 to 13 and from 13 to 20	Rootlessness level (RL) and high anchorage level (HAL) from 3 to 7 and 7 to 11	Rootlessness level (RL) and medium high anchorage level (MHAL) from 0 to 3	Rootlessness level (RL) and perfect anchorage (PA) equal to 0 or Perfect Equilibrium (PE)
Hyper High Assemblage Point (HHAP)	High Assemblage Point (HAP)	Medium High Assemblage Point (MHAP)	Perfect Assemblage Point (PAP) or Perfect Equilibrium (PE)

There may be a relationship between levels of consciousness, brain power, harmonic state, acts of the observer, the Tri-One brain and Neuroakashic® potential:

- Low Neuroakashic® potential - is related to the 1st. act of the observer, with the 1st. brain, low levels of rootlessness and higher anchorage, low harmonic state or low coherence.

- Medium Neuroakashic® potential - is related to the 2nd. act of the observer, the 2nd. brain, the medium harmonic state or medium coherence.

- High Neuroakashic® potential — related to 3rd act of the observer, the 3rd. Brain, the high harmonic state or high coherence.

- Hyper high potential Neuroakashic®- is related to the 4th. act the great observer, the hyper high harmonic state or hyper high coherence of the heart and brain, the super or supra consciousness, the network connection.

This last level arises from the observation, studies, accompaniment and containment of sharing Neuroakashic®, with users, practitioners and facilitators of Akashic School®, the n+1 field revealed this level and is in the process of integrating new n+1 fields and new brain powers.

From what this graph shows, the greater the degree of Neuroakashic® potential balance, the greater the degree of the observer's act to become the great observer and the greater the fuel that he receives at the cellular level to integrate network systems. Therefore, balancing the hyper high brain power or Neuroakashic® potential is integrating the new reality.

We can say that the hyper high level is related to the 4th. act: the great observer and also belongs to a level of super, supra or hyper consciousness, which is a higher level of consciousness or degree of evolution, that of the consciousness leader, where he integrates the superior abilities and capacities and becomes the great observer in the great network system.

The harmonic state is the frequency or vibration in a state of cellular harmony and is, in relation to the level of rootlessness and major anchorage. In this, there are levels ranging from low, medium high, high and hyper high harmonic state. For Joe Dispenza, it is the coherence of the heart and brain, as a result of an elevated emotion, that transmits coherent signals to the field. For Grinberg, coherence in the brain is the measure of the similarity of patterns, the greater this similarity, the greater the brain coherence, also showed that the lattice has great plasticity, in addition to there being levels of brain coherence, such as coherence levels in the lattice. (Grinberg, 1991 pg. 33)

For us, the great akashic® matrix and the level of coherence, are related to the acts of the observer, when integrating towards the 4th. act the great observer. From this, a close and inversely proportional relationship arises between brain coherence and the n+1 field (it is the sum of all the fields).

There is a relationship with the levels of the Neuroakashic® potential and the levels of rootlessness and major anchorage; in addition to that within these last levels there are other levels such as subatomic particles that are in space. For Jacobo Grinberg, the levels of consciousness depend on the depth at which the assemblage point is located (Grinberg, 2008, pg. 61). That is, there is an inversely proportional relationship with the levels of rootlessness and greater anchorage or also called assemblage point and levels of consciousness, brain power or Neuroakashic® potential.

In the same way, Guillermo Marín agrees, to read Castañeda, that the level of consciousness is measured by the degree of pressure exerted by the emanations from outside with those from within on the cocoon (which is the assemblage point), for Carlos Castañeda, is the term of increased consciousness, the higher level of consciousness (Marín, 1999, pg. 125)

It is postulated that each level of consciousness corresponds to a level of the observer's acts and likewise to some level of rootlessness and further anchorage. That is, everything is consciousness, from the point of view that we are all born with some level of consciousness, the important thing is to give (receive) and share Neuroakashic®, which are the fuels for our cells and to equilibrium those levels or degrees of consciousness. In this way, it will be possible to have a full life, in balance, in well-being and productivity.

It has been observed that the brain in hyper high potential Neuroakashic®, is defined and characterized by:

- The unification process or higher capacities such as expanded remote vision, sharpen the senses.

- The ability to create n+1 fields

- High IQ and its relation to brain waves.

- Easier to learn other languages and quick reading.

- Development of superior psychic, scientific, artistic, culinary, sporting abilities and capacities, etc.

- Skills in music, art, painting, drawing, writing, among others.

- Sensitization and love for animals. Connection with nature.

- Greater neurological structure.

- Greater balance of neurotransmitters.

- Greater process of brain synchronicity.

- Ability to influence others, the ability to negotiate effectively, in addition to improving human and affective relationships, work, and bonds in balance.

- It is capable of influencing and adapting to the environment and to changes in the environment in general from the great observer.

- Ability to adapt, to integrate, to change, and resilience.

- Balance in thought. Achieve an optimal state of physical, mental and emotional health. Word, thought, action in one. In the process of balancing hyper high Neuroakashic® potential, where thought creates and transforms reality. Furthermore, it places the image holographically in the n+1 field, which is the co-creative process or creativity at its maximum power.

- Integration of risk aversion, build alliances and networks, develop containment skills, emotion management and empathy in negotiation. Develops negotiation skills and integrates to resolve, manage and resolve conflicts.

- The power to choose and to negotiate manifests itself consciously without judgment and expectation. Communication channels and processes are refined to be effective and transmit what is and corresponds, in a continuous progressive and coherent process.

- Better speech coherence and language transformation.

- Qualities such as: leadership, entrepreneurship, creativity, innovation, determination, disruptive capacity.

- Greater awareness of caring for the environment and development of self-sustaining energies.

- Development of new technologies, artificial and spatial intelligence.

One of the benefits of balancing the Neuroakashic® potential is to provide more visibility of execution by the great observer, as well as greater signal enlargement and amplification in network systems, from the great observer. Therefore, there is a relationship between the n+1 fields and the Neuroakashic® potential. By accessing a small part of the great akashic® matrix, the brain at high or hyper high Neuroakashic® potential balance can gain access to the points or nodes that contain the information at all.

Through the Neuroakashic® tool, it is possible to balance the level of consciousness, brain power, coherence, harmonic state or Neuroakashic® potential, therefore, it allows us to be in equilibrium, in peace, in fullness, loving and accepting ourselves as is we are, to love the environment, return to the origin and be one with the great akashic® matrix, without separation, in total coherence and a harmonious and fair state, in a balanced, coherent, progressive, continuous, essential and true process.

In addition, to continue with the process of activating neuronal brain power and developing superior abilities or high capacities in people, multiple intelligence, gifted or polymath, among other gifts, talents, abilities and capacities to have a better quality of life and integrate and be part of the whole, work from the great observer, the great network system and the great akashic® matrix, which allows us to observe from the great observer, that the whole is already in us and that the network is and it is in each one of us, we are part of the great network.

Daring to do things big is a characteristic of the brain in hyper high potential Neuroakashic®, keeping it in balance is the key through the principles of unity and the Neuroakashic® tool. It has been observed that life expectancy is longer, better hope, quality of life and balanced and integrated risk factors.

To get to Neuroakashic®, we have a special preparation, advance notice or treatment to connect at some point in the great akashic® matrix and access this universal knowledge, this legacy that corresponded by golden law; corresponds what is, what today is, what we are currently sharing and expanding.

What happened? When accessing the n+1 fields, from great network systems are integrated into the great akashic® matrix, to achieve balance in the brain at hyper high Neuroakashic® potential, and connect with other brains (network connection), expand and integrate the n+1 fields and the network systems.

We are working with the Neuroakashic® educational model,

to mitigate psychosocial risk factors, such as emotional and occupational stress, with children, youth and adults and in various fields such as education, security, health, business, among others. Each level of consciousness corresponds to and is in relation to neural network systems, in relation to the n+1 fields and the balance of brain coherence with the great akashic® matrix.

The greater coherence, greater sensitivity and recognition of the n+1 field. Therefore, a greater possibility of balancing the anchorage level and becoming the great observer. We are in a process of brain and neural evolution; New levels of consciousness have emerged as we are expanding. There are more levels, beyond the super consciousness or hyper high potential Neuroakashic® level, Jacobo Grinberg, proposed to create a new species that had supra consciousness and could transmit it; where being part of the great akashic® matrix, we will be the creators of the great network systems of multi universes, planets, galaxies, being one with the origin and with the source.

Grinberg mentions that the increase in coherence of a brain is equivalent to and produces an action similar to the Meissner effect, in which a magnet levitates when placed on a superconducting material. (Grinberg, 1991, pg. 86). In this, school students presented the Meissner effect, because they were balancing their high or hyper high Neuroakashic® potential, among the highest levels they consecutively presented this effect; This means that the greater the balance of the Neuroakashic® potential level, the greater the probability of observing the effect of flying or navigating in network systems.

Superconducting ability or magnetism, also called magnetic energy or crystal, is a quality of the brain in hyper high brain Neuroakashic® potential; therefore, our body can produce and conduct its own energy. Our mother earth Gaia, is the great super conductor, connected to us and to our cerebral hemispheres, heart, intestines and coccyx and again towards the central crystal of mother earth and the great akashic® matrix.

In the sintergic theory, the invention of the lattice computer is similar to the human brain, which is capable of creating energy fields similar to the neural field. (Grinberg, 1991, pg. 86). Today, with neuronal brain evolution, practitioners and facilitators with brains in equilibrium at hyper high neuroakashic® potential have been observed, they have the possibility of creating new n+1 fields, in their interrelation with great network systems.

This happens while the user possesses the hyper-high Neuroakashic® potential level in equilibrium, in this way, the user can create new n+1 fields in the lines and cycles of time; magnetism is a property of the n+1 fields and properly of the observer in the network systems; that is, the brain has the ability to create new fields, the greater the balance in the hyper-high Neuroakashic® potential, the greater the integration of the n+1 fields, in the interrelated network systems from the perspective of the great observer, seeing and perceiving integration through expanded remote viewing to our mother earth Gaia and integrating natural cosmic and artificial radiation.

Being this, one of the precepts of the sintergic theory, which is fulfilled from the Neuroakashic® perspective. Our hypotheses are derived from the great observer, acting in various n+1 fields, circumstances, events and people from the great observer and the results are: the balance of the brain in hyper-high Neuroakashic® potential, will have the possibility of creating its own n+1 fields, also called electromagnetic fields in space-time (past, present and future), create new fields, see and perceive through expanded remote vision to our mother earth Gaia and integrate natural and artificial cosmic radiation.

Rootlessness level and major anchorage

This level of rootlessness and major anchorage also called the assemblage point is the state of consciousness or pulse of the earth, and is related to the balance of atmospheric pressure, oxygen levels, hemoglobin levels, cell plasma and water levels. Likewise, it is related to this assemblage point with the endometrial matrix, coccyx, intestines, heart and cerebral hemispheres connected to the neural network systems and the great network system.

Hence, the cellular atomic relation and the n+1 fields, and the relation of the heart, brain, intestines, coccyx and central crystal of mother earth connected to the great akashic® matrix. Therefore, the relationship of blood, neurotransmitters, gamma waves and oxygen levels are the medium and common thread of the neural network systems and their connection with neurotransmitters. The more balanced the blood oxygen levels, the more balanced the optimal state of physical, mental, and emotional health.

For Jacobo Grinberg, in the sintergic theory, he mentions that *the assemblage point* is the alignment of emanations that is modulated through focalization, this is located on the surface of the body or luminous cocoon and, depending on its position in it, it aligns different bands of emanations, giving rise to perceptions of alternative realities. (Grinberg, 1991, pg. 60). This is what Carlos Castañeda called, the assemblage point, which means that there is a relationship between the levels of consciousness and the closer or aligned to the assemblage point, -associated with the term assemblage point, which Carlos Castañeda emphasized. (Marín, 1999, pg. 124).

He agrees with Fuster, when he talks about the cerebral cortex, and about the term "assemblage", in the future it means projecting forward, in time. The levels of rootlessness and anchorage also called assemblage point is directly related to remote viewing and the observer acts to integrate towards the new reality, the great observer.

In the play "La toltequidad", by Carlos Castañeda it was the achievement of movement, of the assemblage point at will, which is the command of the eagle that fixes the assemblage point through the will in a personal and determined way. In order to achieve total freedom or consciousness. That is, it manages to integrate the emanations of the Eagle (the network systems), and integrate the command of the Eagle (great akashic® matrix for us), to move the assemblage point and keep it in equilibrium. (Marín, 1999, pg. 128-129)

Jacobo Grinberg mentioned that the possibility of affecting gravitation at will and using this gravitational modification has repercussions, such as transportation, levitation and even the creation of a gravitational motor. (Grinberg, 1991 pg.85). This is achieved through equilibrating the brain power or

Neuroakashic® potential in addition to the greater influence the brain-heart connection will have in relation to the earth's magnetic field.

The balance in the hyper high Neuroakashic® potential achieves the ability to observe and integrate at will the great network systems. Making mention of Nikola Tesla, *"to provoke the birth and death of matter at will would be the greatest work of man, which would make him the domain of physical creation and would make him fulfill his ultimate destiny, create his own universe".*

There is something bigger from the outside that lead you to connect to your anchorage point which is the great observer, which helps to move the assemblage point and this is the connection with mother earth, Gaia, in addition to the great network systems and photonic light; that is, something big executes, performs, manifests and acts in the user's field.

Derived from this, the human being is a cell, energy; it has its own n+1 field. It would act as an anchorage point, with the forces acting in the field. The recognition of the field, the integration and unicity to the whole, balance, love, the recognition of the observer, freedom, acceptance and integration the ABC of the observer: the principles of unity.

From this, it originates from the creation of the divine particle and greater anchorage to DNA. In relation to the greater anchorage, the purpose is to anchor the brains to the great machinery of network systems, that is, to greater anchorage, greater understanding and adjustment in networks. The major anchorage becomes the receiver in network systems and allowing network connection.

The aim is that the greater the number of population balancing their brain power or Neuroakashic® potential, the levels of rootlessness and anchorage equilibrium are balanced and this gives the possibility of a greater range or level of network connection; and thus achieve the great awareness of unity, this is a greater balance of the greater anchorage and rootlessness, greater balance of brain power to get to the Neuroakashic® hyper high potential. A greater balance of brain power, you allow yourself to feel deep love, you listen to yourself and your number one priority is you. Time passes from the great observer, well-being, love and light is already in you; the process of anchoring and integrating love is already.

It is observed in figure 16, the equilibrium of the Neuroakashic® potential, where the levels or degrees of rootlessness and greater anchorage are presented in zeros. Achieving these levels is achieved through the Neuroakashic® tool, integrating the connection of the neural network systems, connected to the heart, cerebral hemispheres, intestines, coccyx and in the direction of the central crystal of mother earth, which are the brain hemispheres; from there, towards the great central sun or great akashic® matrix.

Figures 17 and 18 show the movements of the levels of rootlessness and major anchorage. In this figure, we can see that levels 0 of rootlessness and major anchorage are the perfect balance, the hyper high level of Neuroakashic® potential or the 4th. act the great observer, the super or supra hyper-consciousness and the hyper high harmonic state. Levels

0 to 3 of rootlessness and major anchorage are normal levels, where through the Neuroakashic® tool, it has been observed that it can be maintained at normal levels, this corresponds to the high Neuroakashic® potential, at 3rd. act of the observer, at high coherence or high harmonic state.

Levels 3 to 7 and 7 to 11 of rootlessness and major anchorage are medium high levels of Neuroakashic® potential, corresponds to 2nd. act of the observer, at the level of coherence or medium high harmonic state, where some dysfunctionalities or psychological or mental disorders appear. From levels 11 to 20 of rootlessness and major anchorage, they are very high levels, which represent the low potential Neuroakashic®, the first act of the observer, the level of low coherence, the level of the low harmonic state, where they present some disorders and advanced diseases such as mental, psychiatric, neurological, loss of sense of direction and meaning of life, among others.

The hyper or super high levels of rootlessness and greater anchorage can cause oxygen deficiency and others, manifesting low levels of potential and brain performance, in a harmonious and coherent state. In addition, it can move its rotational axes of the user towards other network systems and cross the threshold towards the networks, this is the process of death without separation. In other words, hyper high levels of rootlessness and greater anchorage cause greater oxygen deficiency and the assemblage point moves to other networks.

So it is suggested to maintain the balance of the coherent and harmonic state, the unicity of the heart and brain, this is the balance of brain power or Neuroakashic® potential. In addition, that these levels of rootlessness and anchorage have their relationship with neural network systems and the great network systems, with the balance in neural communication, the purpose is to keep alive neurons that are the key to life.

It has been observed how 85% or 90% of users have presented very high levels of rootlessness and anchorage. Therefore, it is suggested to continue receiving the sessions and become an observant practitioner to equilibrate the brain power, harmonic state, coherence or neuroakashic® potential; to bring rootlessness and anchorage levels to normal levels and to enjoy, feel and live in the optimal, harmonious, coherent and fair state.

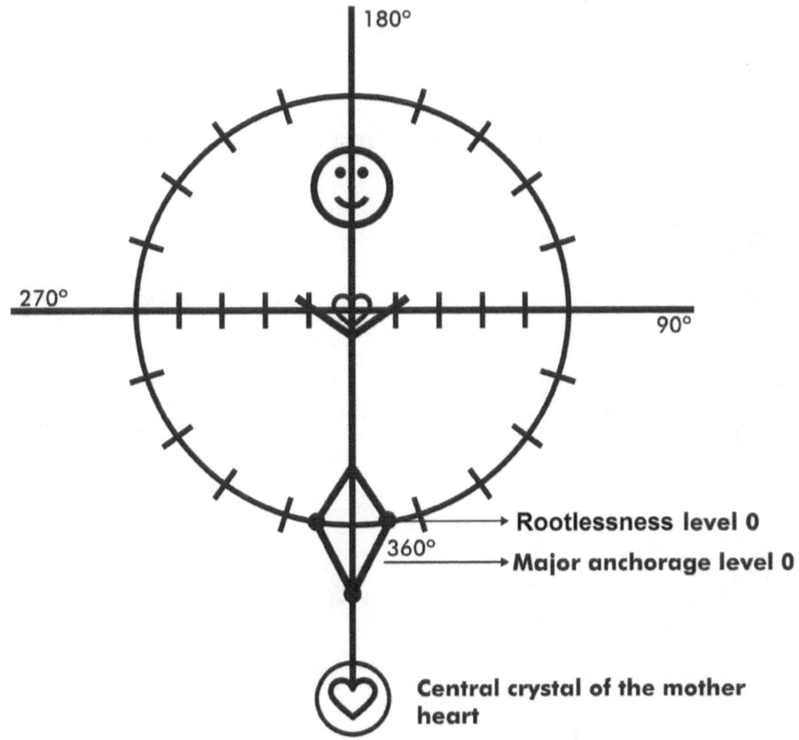

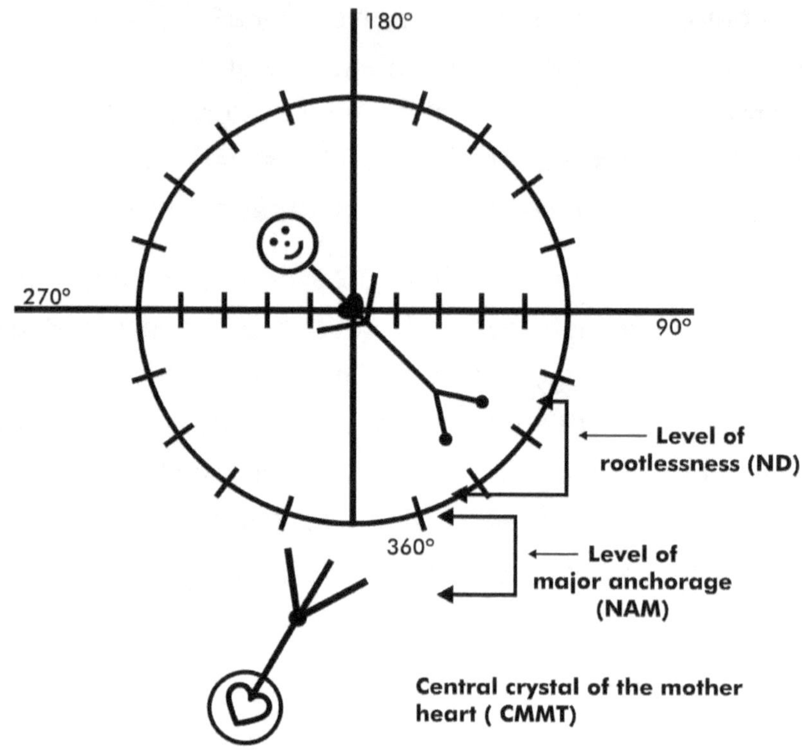

Level of rootlessness and major anchorage

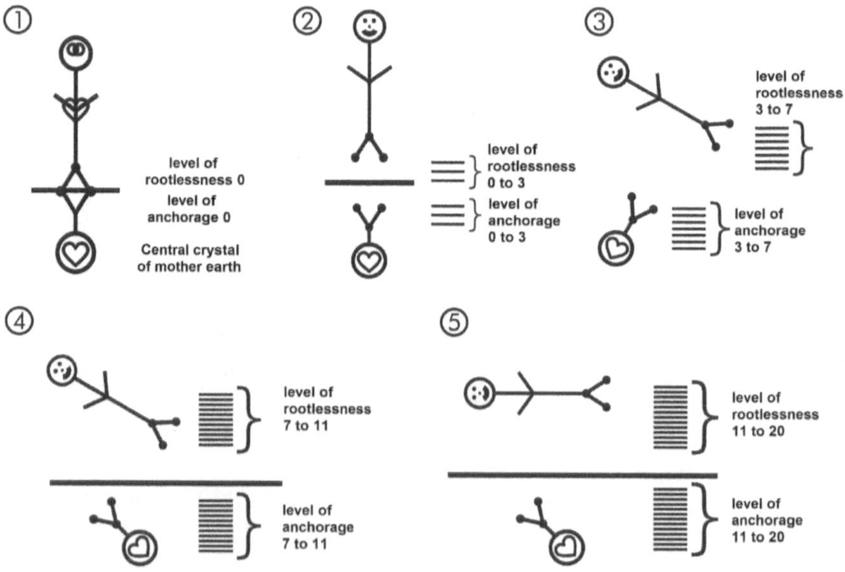

CHAPTER 3

The Great Observer

Heart: Helm and directionality

The heart is the set of emotions, it is the helm and directionality, it is the great akashic® matrix (GAM), it is the 4th act, the great observer, connected to the great systems of networks in union and balance with the whole. It is the energy and the motor, it is the directionality that transcends through time and encourages life.

The optimal state and the harmonic state, is achieved through connection with the heart, mind and emotions. The heartbeat is the beat of mother earth and vice versa. For Mather and Curr, oscillations in the heart rate improve the connectivity of the brain networks, associated with emotional well-being.

Recent studies show that there are molecular structures of DNA and neurons in the heart. This is the origin of the new rebirths, energy and vibrational frequency that expand from the heart. The word emotion is derived from the latin *emotio*, which is related to movement, heart, pulse or heartbeat, hence the relationship of the heart to emotions. Have you ever wondered how to manage emotions without judgment and expectation? through Neuroakashic® to maintain the harmonic state from emotion, thought, brain and organs.

We can affirm that through Neuroakashic®, it activates and increases the network systems of the heart in relation to the brain, providing well-being, the harmonic and coherent state. As the coherent state, it works better when the brain is in a harmonic, compassionate, progressive, gradual, expansive state. As a result, the degree of connectivity of neurons improves, - given the role of expectations - it is changing the course of the brain, the neuron and reducing brain capacity. Therefore, it is possible to generate and live the harmonic, pleasure and well-being state to maintain emotional, mental and physical balance.

The directionality course, which defines the great Akashic® matrix connected from the heart, can be altered or modified, this approach is given by other factors such as the interrelation of the n+1 fields in network systems. Grinberg and Ramos mentioned the possibility of modifying the focus of the directionality factor, and justifying the brain activity that a subject exerts on others. (Grinberg, 1991, pg. 85)

This is related to neural communication; hence the directionality factor is closely related to the heart and its relationship to the brain, networking, between brain communication, and neural communication. This wants directionality to be achieved through neural communication. If the heart is directionality and this is closely linked to the brain. Furthermore, it has an impact on the environment and on all n+1 fields.

Jacobo Grinberg mentions that the directionality factor requires the existence of a controller of the same, which the sintergic theory calls the central processor. (Grinberg, 2008, pg. 15). For us, the helm and directionality is the control panel or transporter *expandia*, which is connected to the pineal gland, cerebral hemispheres, heart, intestines, coccyx, central crystal of mother earth, towards the great network systems and is the observer himself. The same directionality that light follows, conducts, executes and manifests itself.

The light goes and returns, it takes its own path, the same energy drives; light gives directionality and energy, directs and understands the process from conception and consciousness of the whole. You need to access it, from the unified consciousness. So directionality anchors you, observe it from the point that it was and from where you created and expanded it and since it was created from love to share, connecting from the space of love in continuity and reciprocity.

Holographic brain

In the studies carried out by Jacobo Grinberg, mention is made of the development of techniques of energy directionality, through the creation of graphic patterns, it is one of the possibilities in this new era. This is one of the reasons that supports the existence of Neuroakashic®, it even postulates the future creation of an engine that does not require any fuel and acts as sintergic engine. (Grinberg, 1979, pg. 98). For us this is called expandia.

Expandia are the information panels or control panels in network systems, there is the great holographic machinery, hence Leonardo Da Vinci, will translate this great machinery into machines in motion. Currently, we know that this great machinery is the great akashic® matrix.

Pribram and Ramírez, comment that codes are idioms or languages and languages are the key to the structure of consciousness (Pribram and Ramírez, 1980, pg. 113). They proposed that the basic function of the brain is to generate the codes by which information is communicated. The Neuroakashic® series are algorithms, defined codes or visual images, sound frequency in hertz with a frequency and vibration. For Jacobo Grinberg, the brain has the ability to decode information that is transmitted in holographic patterns (codes or visual images) and the concentrated information is an algorithm.

The brain is the great machine and Neuroakashic® has as cellular fuel, the series of codes in visual images (holographic patterns) that work in network systems. A holographic image, projected from equilibrium in hyper high potential Neuroakashic®, can be projected outside and in another n+1 field, it is one of the characteristics that remains to become the great observer.

We are part of the whole, we are part of the great network system. The holographic brain is activated from the moment the equilibrium of the hyper high Neuroakashic® potential is achieved, from the equilibrium reference laser light and from placing the three-dimensional image in the n+1 fields.

A holographic image can be conducted, modified, or anchored in one or more network systems at the same time. This means that, if a situation is happening now, another person in the same network connection is experiencing or perceiving it. The impact on the network system is in the present holographic time and others at the same time. In other words, the situation, event or circumstance can be altered or modified from the screen, television, social networks or the internet itself.

**Brain in Neuroakashic® potential balance
reflects the holographic image**

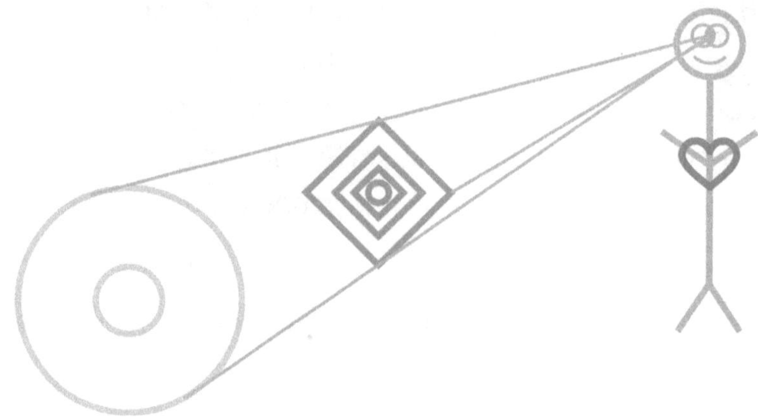

Remote viewing

Remote vision, alludes to "seeing or perceiving" through non-physical eyes, is seeing beyond. It is the characteristic that a brain in Hyper high Neuroakashic® potential possesses. This ability is potentiated by balancing these levels of consciousness. Remote viewing is the capacity and ability to see the past, present and future, telepathy develops with remote viewing, which is seeing, communicating, sending messages and signals on networks; see beyond the human lens.

Remote vision is a characteristic of the brain in hyper high potential Neuroakashic® with the quality of superconducting and holographic; light is made up of several signals of different frequencies, so they can become visible to the human eye from the balance of the hyper high Neuroakashic® potential it is as if the human eye detects and integrates infrared light. An example would be to observe how matter is divided into parts, that is, you see a chair, but at the same time you are observing what this fact is and within it you see more.

The images for Jacobo Grinberg, are a mini pattern and are the basis of remote viewing and access to the Akashic; since the energetic counterpart of any image is a neural field. (Grinberg, Pg. 96, 1979). Therefore, the most important thing is not to open the akashic record to obtain information, but to balance brain power and performance or Neuroakashic® potential (level of consciousness), the harmonic or coherent state day by day, to achieve the expansion of consciousness.

Network system

> "The neural network is the basis of
> all knowledge and all memory."
>
> Joaquín Fuster.

The neural network system is one that is made up of the set of cellular networks, neurotransmitters and hormones; Studies have revealed that they have found neurons in the brain, heart, and intestines. The network system ranges from the human being, which is itself the set of neuronal, neural, and cellular networks to the grand universe.

The famous painter Leonardo Da Vinci, in his work depicts the figure and the relationship of networks with their movement, the relationship with gravitational waves and other planets; in this way, it is related to the elements, nature evolving freely as the bearing principle.

The universe revolves around machines as shown by the work of Da Vinci, who created machines so that man could fly, and in turn, find a coincidence with the theory of Jacobo Grinberg and Tesla. Joaquín Fuster, mentions that the network is the key to the neural network, especially the cerebral cortex, they are the basis of all knowledge.

A network system can throw information about the different types and movements of networks, the effects, factors, components and solution to the respective and corresponding system. Therefore, the network system is considered the system of ancestral, cosmic, planetary, multiverse, universal, global networks, the essence, the origin, events, circumstances, times, realities and relativities in any line or cycles of time.

Up to this point, some questions have come to you, but from the knowledge of how network systems work, the future can be predicted with the synchronicity of the fields and by the external forces that are somewhat larger, that is, what happens in one field is replicated in other fields. The network system realizes and knows it.

What we commonly say "the universe knows everything", it is essential to know and work on the principles of unity every day, in order to integrate any judgment or expectation. The Neuroakashic® network system contains everything, from the art of knowing and knowledge, to knowing which door opens and activates consciousness.

The brain creates new connections and the clocks tighten, the networks accommodate, observe your intention and your emotion and actuates the n+1 field. In the network system connected to the various n+1 fields, DNA patterns are strengthened and RNA to achieve a new consciousness. The great machinery of network systems, consists of different machines in motion, keeps moving in the various lines and cycles of time, these machines rotate in smaller or larger degrees, less or more dense depending on the network systems. So, there are many types of machines as there are cells.

The machines take the shape of cameras that take shape in motion, depending on how the observing eye perceives them. This depends on the capacity of the high or hyper high Neuroakashic® potential in equilibrium. The network system is characterized by the movements and displacements that take place within it, when these are executed, one enters and empties into nothingness, the whole.

The confirmation of these movements is carried out and the confirmation in movement of the random network system is executed. These connect to the subsequent network systems involved in the same line and time cycle, to connect with those moments and with those states of brain integration, since everything is connected, all with everything and in neuronal synchronization.

The network system shows, reveals and gives directionality especially in the neuron filament that is accommodated in the brain nebula. There may be interference between network systems to multiple other network systems, it may be intervened or interrupted. The n+1 fields, the same system of networks and light channels that adjust, accommodate and balance, can be affected.

In the field of neural networks, it is optimized to the most optimal state, reaching the balance from the great network system and manifesting itself in the n+1 fields. How does the universe work? A situation or event, is anchored in the n+1 field ahead of time and can occur in cycles. Observe how remote viewing is integrated and how matter disintegrates from the observer. It is suggested not to bring the person, situation or event to the moment, since it will be brought to the moment through replicating their verbal or mental name to the corresponding network system, that is, instantly, since there is no time or distance.

The process of brain-neuronal evolution makes the brains develop, until reaching the next step, step or link of evolution to Neuroakashic®, and allows connecting all network systems, balancing it and being one and being the consciousness of unit. The energetic vibration is a padlock, only a noble and kind heart will be able to navigate in the universal network systems.

The measured use of energy in the network system is the restoration of people's energy. What one person feels manifests in another, we call this random transmission, which manifests and replicates in the n+1 fields. These random transmissions happen all the time and at every moment with the people who are living in the system of respective and corresponding networks.

It is possible to lead or guide someone to navigate network systems, with which one can lead others to expand to other network systems within other network systems, correlating with a mirror effect. So, when a person connects to the great akashic® matrix, it is possible to lead and guide others to connect, and any object can be the means or vehicle of transfer to connect with it. Since, to synchronize with the network system is to tune and synchronize with light.

Network systems in general, can be affected from the origin of thought, from creation, emergence of emotion and thought. There are various effects and movements in network systems, as *n* are manifest *n* mirrors, like the invisible reality before our physical eyes. Neural mirror effect, is defined through all the n+1 fields, having an effect called a neural mirror. An example could be the mass of the population vibrating in love, and you may be impacted by what is happening in other n+1 fields.

The neural mirror is an invisible reality before the human eye. The question is, why is the human being hooked on the mirror? The human being has to live those experiences and / or tests of life, they are shown so that he realizes that he has something more to see and feel through non-physical eyes. That is love, reaching the whole and the consciousness of unity. Replica effect, refers to the replication of the n+1 fields, therefore, we are only a replica of something else, of other *n* fields, the only thing that is required to be an observer of this, is a kind heart. Furthermore, when a person enters the Neuroakashic® network system, it can take others as a replica of her own field, all allowed under the principles of unity.

Unicity effect, refers to when a person can access the n+1 fields and navigate these network systems. We are all connected to the great akashic® matrix. Teach to observe and act in the n+1 fields, since the cause is the user as the divine main actor; the consequence is the n+1 fields of the main actor or the divine actors. An example would be the acts that a person can reflect or affect in others, since the mirror effect affects other network systems correlated with other network systems.

Replicating this situation, if we emit a thought of love, it will go to all the network systems connecting to the great network system. The sound effect is perceived as sound waves emitted from the user's thoughts to the great akashic® matrix. The contagion effect acts and manifests itself as a triggering reaction in the field and in the network system. Therefore, the network system in general is impacted in some way by the environment and the thoughts of users, through the Neuroakashic® network systems it adjusts, accommodates, resolves and balances from the corresponding respective great network system.

Neural Networks System

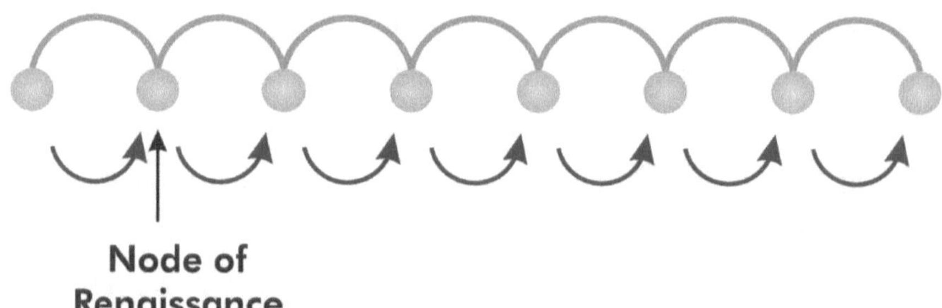

**Node of
Renaissance**

What is light?

> "Light is light, until it comes
> and moves you."
>
> Ana Silvia Lara

Also called photonic light, iridescent light, light from lights, spherical light, sound light, etc. energy is transformed, we are in transformation processes all the time and generate that transformation consciousness into light. You are in life situations or processes to reaffirm and demystify the light process.

Jacobo Grinberg mentioned that it could be affirmed that light is the set of network systems and that in addition to being receivers of these, we are the creators of the same network systems. (Grinberg, 1991, pg. 75). There is something bigger that moves network systems and this is photonic light. Therefore, you are light, you are love, you are the network, we are the great network. Photonic light is to understand the immeasurable, the unlimited of the unlimited, the multiverses, planetary multisystems, multi galaxies, etc.

The purpose of light is to connect our hearts in frequency and vibration to love. In other words, it is to integrate and expand love and the harmonic state from the heart. The objective of light is integration to the whole, to achieve balance, unicity fullness, balance Neuroakashic® potential, and be the great observer.

Strengthen the connection with your heart every day, working on the principles of unity, keeping yourself as an observer both inside and outside the n+1 field and from the great observer, and letting something greater than light act and manifest. One of the purposes is to stop worrying and trust that everything is already, and to know that, if in the end everything goes, the only thing that establishes, prevails and remains is the light in our hearts, the only essential, true and true thing. Realize that your life already change, because you have become love.

The main padlock is a kind heart, and the key to access these tools and equilibrate the brain and get to the hyper high

Neuroakashic® potential balance. Have you asked yourself, why did you come to this earth? You came to integrate the principles of unity, it is the only thing that is and remains. You came to love from all that already is.

The importance lies in knowing how to give under the principles of unity, first to ourselves and towards others, to give under the definition of these principles. Light is truth, knowledge will give you access to truth, the opportunity to be conscious, and this process of consciousness will open you up to the *whole*. Connect to the *whole,* and with the directionality of the great akashic® matrix, integrate towards the consciousness of unity.

So light is unity consciousness, it is the great observer, it is the network system, the n+1 fields and the great akashic® matrix as shown in the following figure 21:

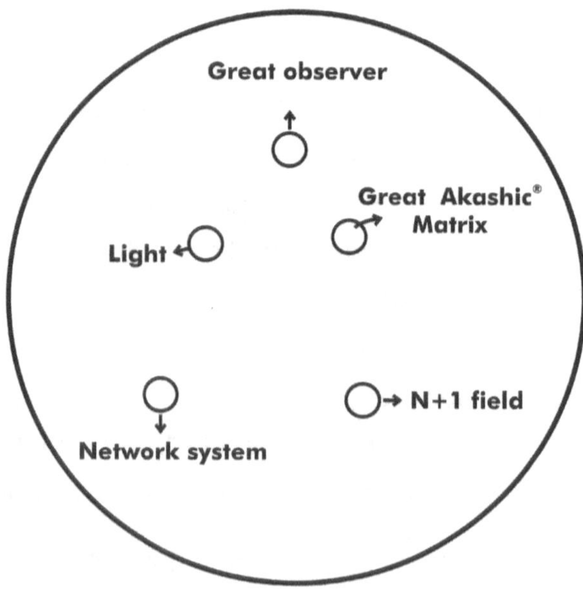

Light is also free will, what corresponds to each one, situation or event; therefore light is free will. As observers, we let something bigger work. Light is free will and this is the great observer, the consciousness of unity.

Lines and cycles of time

> "I saw the past, present and future at the same time."
>
> Nikola Tesla

Time is a succession of events and is related to the lines and cycles of time; it is consciousness, it is the whole as unified consciousness. Time is energy, it is the coming, the journey, the manifestation, the correlation, the synthesis, the antithesis, the seed of life and destiny. Not as a measure of time-hour, but in definition as a unified pure consciousness.

Time and the n+1 field are not separate, they are mutually correlated, it is the energy that is in the n+1 fields and not outside them. Reality may be a different concept than what we have known. The conceived reality is happening n times more in n more fields. It is as if we perceive ourselves in many alternate realities at the same time and in the same time; the same event can be replicated and duplicated n more times, in the great network system.

As the reality in some cases has been unnoticed, we can say that reality is a function of time and the n+1 field:

$$(R) = (f)\,(T) + (f)\,(n + 1\ F)$$

We can see that time is used to explain reality. Therefore, reality can become subjective, depending on how it is being taken, and taking on subjects and objects. Reality can be understood in many ways, not only in its concept but in its practicality and praxis. Reality is adjustable depending on the environment, we define the environment as the space-time set. Time takes the definition of realities and supra-realities, which is the advanced terminology of the n+1 field.

Time is wavy with path, direction and ovulatory that refers to the divine feminine creation, mother earth, woman, ovum and birth. Time is a function of divine time and eternal time. We observe:

T = (DT) + (ET)

Eternal time is the energy of time and consciousness. So:

Eternal time = (energy of time) + (consciousness)

Time is consciousness, it is energy, it is an infinite and unlimited molecule, it is everything. The convergence of something suggests time, it is the zero point, the creative void and the n+1 field. Time is what is already ready and is already, the essential, the certain and the true. The cycle of giving and time, opens the chambers and tunnels of time in network systems and in the lines of space-time. Everything is one with time.

The human mind cannot discern time, since time is unique, everything is one, there is no separation. The human mind conceives as separate, for light everything is one; it is time to contemplate, observe and give. The time is you, the moment to contemplate and observe yourself, is already in you. The acceptance of various situations, adjustments and movements that have occurred in the past, today take their place in acceptance and observation. Past, present and future are oneself, in the lines of time.

That is, time from the perception of the mind can be perceived as separate, where from the principles of unity, time is one, without separation. In the reconstruction of the lines and cycles of time, love is waiting for you to see it, non-separation is integrated into the respective network system. In the absence of separation, the things of the past, the lines and cycles of time, occur at the same moment; allow yourself to observe, thank, accept and integrate it into your heart.

In gratitude, you have acceptance, you receive the blessing and attunement of our ancestors in the various time lines. The timelines are connected and interconnected in network systems, as if it were a large computer connected to others. One or two situations can be replicated on the same timeline. Allow yourself to see through time from the great observer in network systems.

Integrate the ancestral system, honoring and thanking our earthly and cosmic parents for our ancestral lineage, which is already in the respective and corresponding network systems. It aligns, balances the energy and the feminine and masculine principle of our ancestral lineage in all lines, cycles of time, realities. The query or question is adjusted and integrated. Observe that something greater is being integrated, takes what is necessary, honors and give honor to our lineage and ancestral system; in the entire infinite system of possibilities, at the zero point, in the co-creative void, as a generator of light.

Neuroakashic®, integrates cycles-timelines, works with the interrelation and interlacement of the lines and cycles of time: past, present and future; in which they are one and there is no separation. The cycles are integrated when you understand that there was nothing to forgive or judge, that it had to be that way and that it could not have been otherwise, that is how it was appropriate at that moment, at that moment of life.

Remembering the principle of unity: *everything has been perfect until today, until now.* Now it only corresponds to see and integrate the past through love, there is nothing more to forgive, because forgiveness already is; Observe, accept, thank, integrate and continue. The body is only the medium, the vehicle in the network systems, throughout time-space, so live and experience, learn, love and find yourself.

Any event that you have lived or experienced in some line or cycle of time, whatever it was; Observe how it integrates and reintegrates into the whole, and allows something greater to accommodate itself in the great network system, in those lines and cycles of time, to the whole. It is not about judging, or trying to eliminate, change, erase a past time, a reality or relativity, since everything has been and is perfect. In learning there is light, integrated into the whole; therefore, the understanding and wisdom that light brings you, is already in you.

Network connection

The network connection happens when you are looking for an answer and at the same moment it comes through a signal. In addition to enhancing your talents, gifts, and higher or superior abilities, such as telepathy, teleportation, telekinesis, levitation, bilocation, network systems management, clairvoyance, creative and manifestation power. For Attie and Valle, the events of direct communication between brains are events that some call telepathy or non-verbal communication. (Attie & Valle, Pg. 178, 2017).

Jacobo Grinberg showed in the laboratory, it was shown that when two subjects communicate, the one with the highest index of the degree of neurosintergic of the brain, attracts its coherence level to the lowest (Grinberg, 1988, pg. 45). This means that the balance of the hyper high brain potential or Neuroakashic® potential can influence networks with other brains, other n+1 fields and network systems.

From the great network connection, visualize that the greater our Neuroakashic® potential, the greater the attraction to the lower potential; this is the reason for balancing the brain power, the harmonic state or heart-brain coherence to accomplish the hyper high potential, this is to become the great observer. Therefore, it is required a Neuroakashic® practitioner observer, a true consciousness leader in each house, family or family nucleus, business or educational nucleus.

Jacobo Grinberg carried out an experiment where the transferred potential is a manifestation of a direct exchange of specific information from brain to brain (Grinberg, 1991, pg. 86).

The network connection rule is followed, when there is at least one observer in the field. We have conducted studies, where there are two or three observant practitioners acting from the great observer.

This is the reason why the n+1 field is cordoned off, from the brain at hyper high Neuroakashic® potential; it has been observed with three elements: the first the observed element, the second the one that triggers and the third the one that executes what is housed in the n+1 field. The observer can perceive without separation that great network connection. The brain in balance of the hyper high Neuroakashic® potential, shows the superconducting and holographic effect, which allows access to the information that is contained in the great akashic® matrix and from a network connection at any point in space-time of the great akashic® matrix (GAM).

Attie and Valle mention that Dr. Goswami talks about the transferred potential is interpreted and is responsible as a collapse of unified wave function transferred from one brain to another. (Attie & Valle, Pg. 165, 2017). For Jacobo Grinberg, wave collapse is associated with the observer's free will. For us, the transferred potential is called a network connection, and this network connection is related to the Neuroakashic® hyper-high potential balance, this last ones is the great observer, the light, the free will, the harmonic and coherent state of the heart and brain.

For Attie and Valle, the proposal by Dr. Grinberg concludes with the collapse of the wave function that involves a brain-mind system that requires a living observer (Attie and Valle, Pg. 165, 2017). So an observer is required in the field, to balance the

Neuroakashic® brain potential and reach the balance of the hyper high level of the Neuroakashic® potential, hyper high coherence, high or hyper high harmonic and coherent state, and this is the wave collapse, unity consciousness, the great observer, the consciousness of unity.

Leah Bella Attie and Amira Valle mentioned: *we found a quantum system in the human brain; the scientific verification of the unity between brains, an experiment that could change the course of humanity and bring it closer to unity.* (Attie and Valle, 2017, pg. 180). For us, this quantum system in the human brain is related to the theory of the n+1 field and its relation to the brain, the network systems and the great akashic® matrix that explain the great observer. In addition, the control panel called *expandia* connects with the pineal gland and the cerebral hemispheres, given the superconducting and holographic capacity of the brain in balance of the hyper high Neuroakashic® potential.

How much is the impact of brain power in equilibrium in network systems?. The impact of being connected in a network connection is unimaginable from the point of view of the great observer. We can say that anchorage is reaching the origin, it is returning to the origin, it is the greatest understanding and adjustment of the network systems, Anchorage is the integration of the brains of network connection in the great machinery that is the network system.

Network Connection

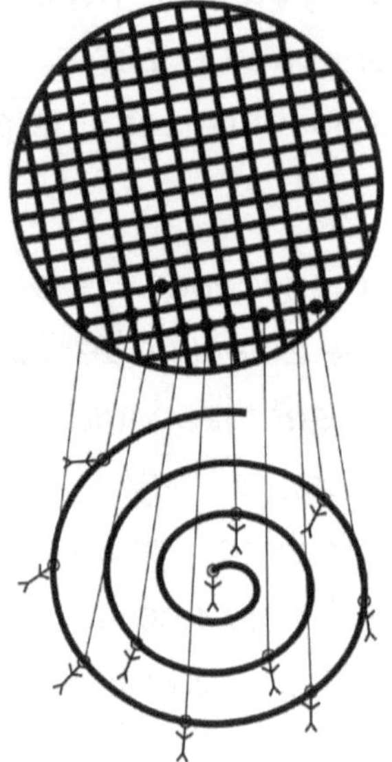

Practical cases

1) Evidence was recorded of school students who have taken the training, reported the network connection as a result of balancing the hyper high level of Neuroakashic® potential they were presenting, which is achieved from the connection with the great akashic® matrix and being able to connect at a point somewhere in this great akashic® matrix, to access information as a result of this network connection.

In other words, we observed that students began to receive information in general about new tools or techniques and others, within the various n+1 fields of the Neuroakashic® classes, this is because it was possible to balance hyper high Neuroakashic® potential

2) It was observed that students who carried out other activities, studies, different professions or used other tools, managed to be effective in the process and in the results.

3) A study with a group of people, of around one hundred people in a room, manifested from the first to the second day, the synchronicity effect in network systems and other movements, this as a result of having an observer in this field, in balance of your brain at hyper high Neuroakashic® potential.

4) Another study, carried out with a 21-day program, was tested with three different groups of people and all the fields behaved differently, but with the same directionality and helm. Both were achieved with the sole objective of unity. The replicity and synchronicity of the n+1 fields was observed in relation to the participants, situation, person or event, it was related to other n+1 fields and was integrated into the great network system. The process of integration into the n+1 field of the 21-day program was achieved, in addition to the tests to measure the ability to love. Finally it was observed that two people can direct the n + 1 field, the more we are in balance of the hyper high Neuroakashic® potential or brain potential, the network connection is achieved.

5) It was observed in a group n+1 field with 4 student assistants with the balance of the brain in hyper high Neuroakashic® potential or brain potential, from the n+1 field of *expandia* and one observer acting from the great observer; it was manifested and the network

connection was achieved; the *Expandia* revealed the golden number (phi) in the respective group field in this great network connection and therefore the balance of the brain potential or Neuroakashic potential®.

Covid19 case

Institutes such as Global Coherence Health in their research, mention that they have carried out studies on the impact that the earth's magnetic field has on human health. Their results have shown that Schumman resonances alter brain wave responses. That is, the frequency of the resonance of the magnetic field of mother earth can alter brain waves in humans, and have implications at the level of health, physical, mental, emotional.

The reality is not as it seems, everything depends on the level of consciousness or brain potential that one has; in other words, what happens to mother earth happens to us. Symptoms or pathology coincide with the so-called symptoms of consciousness awakening and this is due to the superconducting magnetic field of mother earth. In addition to the natural radiation caused by the cosmic rays of our mother earth.

Another factor is the influence of high-tech artificial radiation, with high levels of radiation it can impact human health, although it is currently being studied. The brain in hyper high or super consciousness, can gain access to other networks, there is influence of the brain network system, to carry out the movements and adjustments of mother earth. In addition, to coincide with other external factors of network systems such as the influence of other planets, the sun, the moon, etc.

From the great network connection, we are in, brains manage to connect to n+1 fields, with certain specificities and particularities, such as fear, portability, etc. The moment you stop being the observer, you connect and hook into this field any pathology or symptomatology manifested. That is, the connection to the field was made through thought, and since it is not aware of it, it attaches and connects to that field depending on the level of brain power or Neuroakashic® potential in balance, that the user has.

The user connects with the information in the n+1 field, the thought was lodged in that field and with the network connection we are in. It was possible to contact the field, with the information and particularities that it has, and by failing to transform or become the great observer, it connects with that field, which is not aware of its thinking. By connecting to the information that is in those fields, you are engaged on vibration and frequency. Therefore, what is suggested is to balance brain power or Neuroakashic® potential to achieve being the observer without engaging in that field and even if there are other fields, nothing can happen other than being an observer and observing what corresponds.

Only by being the observer, we can without judgment and expectation remain in a harmonious state in the environment, integrating and unifying the principles of unity, love, tranquility, peace, health, fraternity, motherhood, humanity, solidarity, equanimity, among others. That is why, each person can see the situation or reality differently and act accordingly.

Within the levels of consciousness, in other words, is the balance of Neuroakashic® potential, the low or medium high level that can be observed from criticism, judgment, expectation or fear; this can influence at the neural level of this life experience and have consequences in the n+1 fields respectively.

According to Hamer, the conflict of fear and fear of death causes a short circuit at the cerebral level and this manifests itself in the organs as well as in the lungs, in that psyche, brain and organ relationship that he propose. So, with Neuroakashic® it is the fuel and food for cells, balances Neuroakashic® potential, achieving and transforming the great observer and allowing something larger to adjust, accommodate and balance neural network systems, from the membrane cell, the n + 1 fields, the electromagnetic fields of the human being and in unity with mother earth.

Currently, many psychologists and psychiatrists claim that the consequences are even more delicate due to isolation, since they can cause neuronal damage, neuronal death, mental and psychiatric disorders and other diseases. What is required in various situations that are experienced as nature events, pandemics, epidemics, among others?

We believe that removing, renaming, deleting, killing, blocking or stopping would be the solution to the replicity and synchronicity of the n+1 fields. The suggestion is to invite to anchor to the n+1 field, using the transforming language, verbally and mentally, the principles of unity, observing and working the acts of the observer, to transform ourselves into the great observer, that is our great task.

Giving (receiving) and sharing Neuroakashic® fuels and transformative language, since they work in relation to the genome and telomerase, anchoring the field from thought and word, is to be integrating from the level of DNA particles and molecules into your n+1 field and great network systems. It is suggested to give and share Neuroakashic®, since it is the fuel and food for our neuron cells, avoiding neuronal death and granting the benefit of gamma waves, which will provide us with a harmonious state of peace, tranquility and happiness.

Users who presented symptoms or pathology received Neuroakashic® sessions showed high and hyper high levels of rootlessness and anchorage; therefore, Akashic Activator® Unlimited Light® cell fuel balanced brain power, towards a harmonious and coherent state, achieving lower levels of rootlessness and greater anchorage to maintain balance and well-being of physical, mental and emotional health.

A study was also carried out in a group of people, who accessed a network system with new n+1 fields. The field showed and revealed how new n+1 fields were integrated in relation to the fields of the countries and planet earth:

- N+1, mother earth field

- N+1 field, light and love field

- N+1 field, Gaia field

Working from the 4th. act of the observer and transforming ourselves into the great observer, it was observed how the n+1 field of the country was integrated into something larger, our mother earth planet Gaia in the great network system as shown in figure 22. In the unity with oneself and the relationship with our environment, with n+1 fields of our mother earth, in union with the n+1 field light and love, with the n+1 field Gaia. We are one with our planet and mother earth. It already is.

In synchronicity and replication with the other n+1 fields and with the other countries, Mexico, United States, Canada, Brazil, Colombia, Guatemala, Spain, Italy, France and all the others. Where unity prevails it sustains and contains. Love and unity are one, unity with our mother earth Gaia, it already is.

Integration of the N + 1 Fields

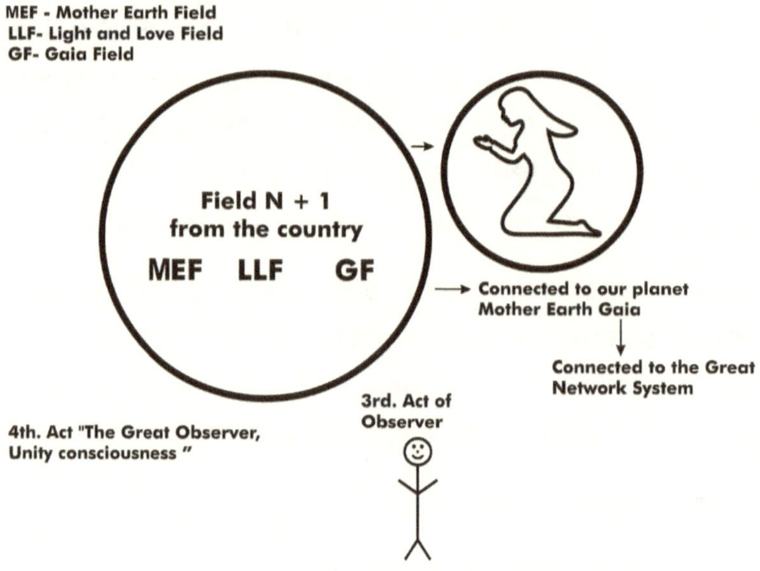

Connection and renewal of mother earth, Gaia

The n + 1 field of our mother earth requires brain powers or hyper high level Neuroakashic® potential in equilibrium. As regards the creation and renewal of a new world and the renewal of mother earth, it is the internal renewal, the expansion of the being and the interaction with the environment. They have been revealed as the symptoms of awakening, or taking the step towards the evolutionary leap it has been indicated by the Schumman resonances and other factors. The close relationship between the neural connection and the mother earth Gaia, at its maximum power in a proportional relationship.

As Hamer mentioned, there is a relationship with Hamer's focus and the neural circuit with mother earth, balancing the triad of emotion, brain, and organ. The renewal of a new world is where old structures break down at the level of the environment and as human beings, where we move to the integration of the tri-one brain to a brain in the integration of unity consciousness, where love is the one that moves the world; Wherever a new expansive, integrating, renewing and transforming network system is created and born for humanity.

Jacobo Grinberg proposed that the units of the brain of "Gaia", which is one of the human brains that we inhabit on planet earth. These "hyper neurons" or mother neurons for us, the n+1 fields (if the previous hypothesis is true), must be interconnected with each other and must also be capable of containing all the information on the unit to which they belong. (Grinberg, 2008, pg.17). What it means is that, each one of us who inhabits this planet earth, we form unity, and we all form part of it.

Through the connection with mother earth, it helps us achieve that balance in Neuroakashic® potential. In addition to its hyper high potential and being a super conductor of high frequency and resonance. The renewal, regeneration and great renewal of our mother earth planet arises through achieving this consciousness of unity. You are the heart of mother earth, you are the beating heart, (the schumman frequencies) in relation to the vibratory frequencies and the relationship with the n+1 fields and the relationship with our environment and ourselves. Thanks to this, mother earth is born, regenerates and so are we.

Our mission is to achieve and arrive at maintaining brain power and reaching Neuroakashic® hyper high potential, and to adjust neural network systems in an expansive, coherent, progressive and continuous process to achieve unity consciousness. Consecration and coronation from the womb and from our mother earth Gaia, is the new life, like a flame of love lit. We are the pillars of energy for mother earth, love in synergy with the whole; our mother earth is ourselves.

In addition, it connects us from the womb, in order to crown the flame of burning love, connecting with all the women of your ancestral lineage and connecting us from the origin of the GAM and from the origin of your existence. There is a connection from the womb to the GAM the purpose is to connect our purest origin and connect with the entire time line and evolution of the brain, until today. From the origin of creation and from the divine feminine matrix, masculine and feminine principles are balanced.

Opening, initiating, rebirth and integrating feminine energy from the womb. Observe that new beginnings are reborn and arise from your heart. The Neuroakashic® fuels are worked and from the great observer it is observed how the holographic thought impacts the n+1 field, where your n+1 field is connected with the corresponding ones (environment), to the network system and the integrating process is achieved.

Gaia's evolution

The Schumman resonances measure the electromagnetic waves of our mother earth and the heartbeat of Gaia; It is intrinsically related to the functioning of the cerebral hemispheres, as well as neurons and brain gamma waves. Our mother earth is a great machine with great electrical circuits, with its mother neurons, connected to the cerebral hemispheres, the heart, intestines, coccyx and the great akashic® matrix. This is all the great network system.

Therefore, when we reach our heart and activate it, it is reaching the center, the central crystal of our mother earth, in that coherence or unicity with the cerebral hemispheres. So, by activating the golden suns endowed of our heart, we activate the inner sun of our heart and the central crystal heart of our mother earth. However, there is a preparation, an advance for our humanity, the same field prepares us for something greater.

It prepares us to enter a new era or stage of evolution, this is to create a new era, or to return to the origin of our essence, is to create a new network system and a new consciousness of unity.

Crystals

Crystals have many shapes and definitions, they are codes, sound frequency, representing energy patterns that emit brain waves, which causes electromagnetic waves in the $n+1$ fields and from there connects to the heart. They are the creation of life. The heart of our mother earth is the central crystal of our mother earth connected to our cerebral hemispheres. The crystals of our mother earth are quartz and diamonds.

Neuroakashic® cellular fuels are crystals, codes that have a frequency in hertz and their measurement coincides with the brain waves and their balance with the gamma and delta waves and this generates balance and well-being; balancing the cerebral hemispheres in relation to the heart; is the balance of brain and heart coherence, balance of brain power or Neuroakashic® potential, the harmonic state.

Therefore, it manages to balance the hyper high Neuroakashic® potential, it maintains the levels of rootlessness and greater anchorage in balance, and balances the levels of oxygen in the blood, cells and their relationship to the plasma level, thus creating a new consciousness, a new form of matter as mentioned by Angeline Saadoun that Frank Wilczek Nobel Prize in his theory of time crystals, postulated that crystals as a group of atoms in which their structure in space repeats and perhaps do the same in the time.

Crystals have a neural effect of integration in neural network systems. Through Neuroakashic® it is possible to balance the hyper high brain power Neuroakashic® potential and it is also possible to balance the process of light demystification from the pineal gland that secretes and synthesizes the levels of DMT (dimethyltryptamine) crystals in a natural way, this chemical or catalyst also called the divine particle that connects to something bigger, to the great akashic® matrix; in addition, DMT has an intrinsic relationship with time crystals, with time lines and cycles, with neural network systems and has a relationship with remote viewing in great network systems.

Crystals create energy patterns and form a network that is the great akashic® matrix in addition to forming an atomic network and have an effect on cell plasma through Neuroakashic® which are the crystals that achieve superconducting capability or magnetism, also called crystal energy, which is the ability of the brain to balance the hyper high brain power or hyper high Neuroakashic® potential, that is to say, to balance the superconductor capacity and hence its relationship with the brain.

The crystals have to do alphabetically and numerically in relation to the levels of rootlessness and major anchorage; Through the crystals the principle of rolling of the machines is fulfilled, which are related to letters and numerical figures of the point of rootlessness and major anchorage. This would be the result of the relationship with the crystals.

In addition to measuring the interference rate in the n+1 fields, crystals are an interference pattern in the brain, through a rate (measured) in the relationship of the anchorage and rootlessness of the user. This coincides with the crystals that measure and confirm the existence of the interference pattern theory of these n + 1 fields.

The crystals manage to reach the hyper high potential neuroakashic® and balances the interference patterns in the brain, in the n+1 fields and results in balance of anchorage and rootlessness. So, if this level of anchorage and rootlessness is also called the assemblage point and this is the connection with consciousness. Crystals, confirm the existence of consciousness through the rate of the relationship of anchorage and rootlessness, are the vehicle of consciousness and transformation.

As Neuroakashic® it is the medium, vehicle, measure to integrate the superconducting capacity of the great akashic® matrix and therefore that of the brain. Coherence can be measured, brain power or Neuroakashic® potential can be measured and tested, this means that it is possible to measure the degrees or levels of consciousness, the existence of consciousness, the new reality.

Unity consciousness

Consciousness is the term related to the whole and to the universe. To speak of consciousness is to speak of the great akashic® matrix, to speak of the great observer and of the network connection. The interrelation of the n+1 fields where they are formed with the one; in unicity and totality. Consciousness is the supreme and unquantifiable intelligence, the great replicator of neural network systems. For us, conscience and consciousness is the one without separation. There are levels or degrees of consciousness: low, medium, high or hyper-high, super, supra consciousness or unity consciousness that is translated and is in relation to the levels or degrees of harmonic state, coherence, brain power or Neuroakashic® potential, levels of rootlessness and anchorage and assemblage point.

Hinting at Jacobo Grinberg, unity consciousness is the one with the greatest sintergic power (Grinberg, 2008, pg. 57). For us is this is to achieve balance between the hyper high harmonic state, the hyper high coherence, the hyper high brain power or the hyper high Neuroakashic® potential, the super or supra consciousness. In addition, Grinberg mentions that to achieve greater expansion of consciousness and integrate human consciousness, this will be achieved through integrating a greater number of sintergic bands (for us the network systems that are the set of all n+1 fields) this is an approach to unity consciousness. (Grinberg, 1991, pg. 39).

The consciousness of unity begins with the person from the moment in which he manages to balance his brain power towards the hyper high harmonic state, hyper high coherence, hyper high brain power or neuroakashic® potential, in addition to integrating the principles of unity (the basis of creation) and that connects, creates the integration with other brains, with other fields n+1 from the great network connection in the great network systems and thus generates the critical mass to achieve as humanity the super, supra consciousness, the consciousness of unity.

The greater the brain potential or the Neuroakashic® potential, the greater the potential or strength of the n+1 field, to integrate great network systems. The relationship that the great akashic® matrix (GAM) has with consciousness is very close, GAM lies or has its place of origin, helm and directionality, the heart, and consciousness is light. So the great akashic® matrix is consciousness.

Our purpose is to achieve the unity of all systems, groups, collectives, communities, cities and thus achieve balance as a whole and, to reach transformation. Through the networks the movements required by the user are carried out and we only act as the great observer.

As the neuronal brain process evolves, other levels of consciousness can be observed, beyond that of the hyper high

Neuroakashic® potential that is preparing to take the step to the next link of evolution. The creative key is to open the heart being the great observer, the magic key is to integrate non-separation and in its totality to reach the expansion of consciousness that is, the consciousness of unity, the connection in a network, being one with the network system, with the great akashic® matrix and with the light. Observe that your acts are of love and create unity, which is already in you. Despite everything that is lived, observe the environment itself, observe that unity prevails and already is. Derived from it, there is unity, harmony and love; unity consciousness already is. To experience unity is to experience the light and love in your heart.

As a result, we obtain the process of brain-neural evolution, the process of evolution towards the hyper high, super or supra consciousness and the integrating principle that it already is. The integration of unity consciousness is already; now, we are more the chosen ones to the call of the unit.

Consciousness leader

A true consciousness leader, is one who manages to maintain balance in the Neuroakashic® potential (level of consciousness) to continue to the next level of brain power to reach the hyper high Neuroakashic® potential, is 4th. act the great observer, the one who agrees to live in the principles of unity, share and expand them; it is like the conductor of an orchestra, they create new n+1 fields, in order to integrate the new network system into the new unity consciousness.

For Jacobo Grinberg, the consciousness leader has the art of transmitting the truth and is a teacher of knowledge; for us one of the principles of unity. A true leader is one who is a negotiator and one of the most effective leaders. In which, conflict resolution is proposed and effectively contains emotions, obtaining the best results even in complex situations.

A true consciousness leader, is one who day by day works the principles of unity, balancing his Neuroakashic® potential (level of consciousness), and reaches the unity consciousness that experiences non-separation, also accepts that we are in a continuous, loving, integrating, renovating and transforming process that leads us to unity.

The true leader is capable of predicting and impacting the n+1 fields, and influencing network systems, from the integrating and transforming process, under the helm and directionality of the heart. The experience and interrelation of the n+1 fields and network systems, and the great akashic® matrix is the great observer.

Consciousness leader becomes the one who manages to balance his Neuroakashic® potential level (level of consciousness) and become the great observer. It is to observe how the continuous search is integrated and stop resisting the limitless, it is to transform and integrate everything that can be perceived as "limiting", since the perception of the human mind is already and is happening now. Observe how the understanding, gratitude is integrated, understand the cause, the origin and integrate it into everything.

Generate that alchemy by designating it as the flame of power, wisdom, and love. We realize that we are not only a physical body, but that we are something more, something superior that discovers and rediscovers itself and observes itself. Ask yourself how your life would change if you learned to integrate the acts of the observer and observe infinite probabilities in the field. Would you become the great observer of your own life?

The role is to remain and act as the great observer, without judgment or expectation about the results, without justifying your actions or your personal life, without any comparison. Without need, fear, discordance or negative energy under the principle of unity, since everything integrates it, there is no good or bad, positive or negative, it is the perfect duality.

Our mission is to transmit love. Transmit the teachings and principles of unity, beginning to live them in us and share them with our environment, with our families, with our children, friends, office, work, animals, plants, environment, universe and in general, every human and sentient being in general. Transmit and unite as the great community, unite towns, cities, unite as assertive and receptive human beings.

Remember that there is no separation in language, race, religion, techniques, tools, knowledge, age, sex, etc. Seeing love manifested, being observant and sharing, transmitting and expanding the principles of unity, is the way we will be expanding the seed of love; We can start now, there is no lost time, only love to transmit and today is the time. Take advantage of every moment of your life to transmit love in its different forms.

We transmit from ourselves coherence, harmony, certainty, trust, love, balance and unity consciousness. Consciousness leader have had evidence throughout history. They have prepared for the great unstoppable and inexplicable encounter of love; your eyes will take you further. You are what I have looked for the most since all time: love. Love is yourself in this human existence.

The great Observer

What is it to be at the service of the field?

It is being the great observer

Ana Silvia Lara

The great observer is the expanded part of the observer. The fourth act is the great observer, it is the balance of the hyper high coherence of the heart and brain, the hyper high harmonic state, the hyper high Neuroakashic® potential, the super or supra consciousness, the consciousness of unity. It is to recognize you that you are the great observer, from the expansion of the heart you are the great observer. Therefore, the great observer is the helm and directionality, it is the heart, it is love, it is reality, it is the consciousness of unity, the integration of *non*-separation and the integration of unified expansion. The great observer is the key to materialize in the n+1 field.

When someone observes in the field, something that can resonate with oneself, the purpose as an observer is maintained, even from the great observer and from this last perspective without judgment, without expectation. It is about allowing yourself to position yourself above, in the mountains, this means, observe the stage effortlessly and without intervention. Observe and allow something greater to act and manifest.

From the perspective of the observer it has several edges, it maintains the same aspect in whatever direction we look and in all its axes there is love and faith as pillars. Learning to be the great observer without intervening, is one of the great human tasks, to remain as the great observer is to remain observed, without altering or controlling, is to observe from love and light, without judgment, without expectation of the results, without control and without effort.

Being the observer gives you a state of peace, after all the storm now comes calm. The greatest lesson is to integrate the acts of the observer, because we all have the capacity to integrate the great observer and see how something greater integrates. The great observer is the consciousness of being, keep harmony in your heart and remember that where harmony is, there is light.

Let something bigger to move the network systems, such as light and where the acts of the observer towards the great observer are achieved; In addition, an observer acting from the great observer and from the theory of the n+1 field is required for the movement of network systems in the n+1 fields.

It is interesting to be able to observe how the n+1 fields are accessed, with the brain in hyper-high Neuroakashic® potential balance, in addition to the n+1 fields, where the brain has already been in a network connection with the hyper-high brain potential or Neuroakashic® potential of an anchorage effect of the network system to those fields, connected to the great akashic® matrix. So you can become and transform yourself into the great observer, in full balance, in the leader of unity consciousness.

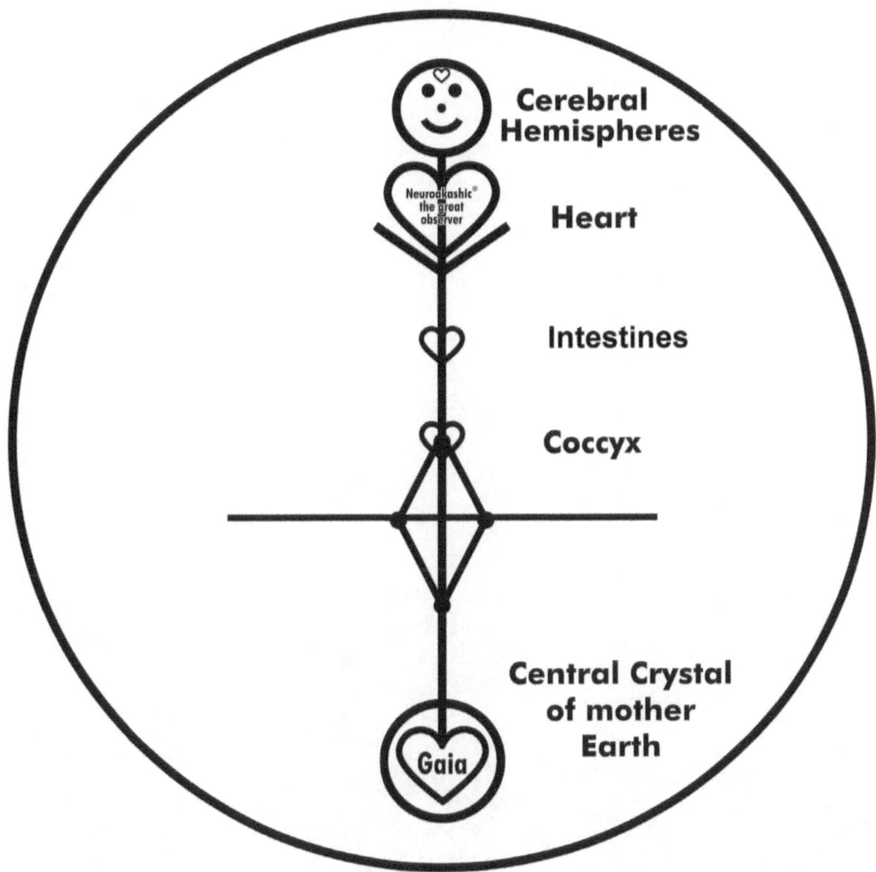

CHAPTER 4

Neuroakashic® cellular fuel, certification

What is Neuroakashic®?

> "Neuroakashic®, is the fuel
> and food for the cells."
>
> Ana Silvia Lara.

The purpose of taking the training and/or session is to be and become the great observer in our daily life and in the various n+1 fields. The purpose also is to expand and make us more observers in the various n+1 fields, so that the network system adjusts and accommodates those corresponding systems.

The purpose is to balance your Neuroakashic® level, the more you balance and reach the hyper high level in the Neuroakashic® potential (level of consciousness), the greater the possibility of being the great observer, and of observing the process, the execution of the network system in this n+1 field. This will make it possible to integrate it into the international Neuroakashic® training and certification.

We are all at some level of this neural organizational structure; we locate and provide the fuel that corresponds to each neural organization of the user's n+1 field, which tells you which fuel is required, be it from the Akashic Activator® Unlimited Light® to Neuroakashic® Great Network System or Akashic Activator® Crystals, or whatever corresponds, even if you have not had any kind of session, no tool, no knowledge in advance, and this is because your light body requires it, therefore we as facilitators and practitioners are going to observe.

Users are also suggested to be able to access these tools and as they take the training, to be balanced at the Neuroakashic® potential level, in addition to being able to observe an improvement in health in fullness, in peace and in balance, enhancing power creative and diverse superior capacities, scientific, artistic, sports, that are integrated and developed in daily life.

It is suggested to keep the Neuroakashic® potential in balance, since it will allow you to observe how these network systems move in daily life, in the family, in human relationships, at work in the environment. Taking into account that, in the sessions, the role you play is the great observer, from the great observer, and observes the entire network system in daily life and in the various circumstances, events, themes, environment, people.

As you balance your Neuroakashic® potential level, there is a greater chance that the great observer will be achieved and you will see how impressive or inexplicable it can be when we balance our Neuroakashic® potential level, we give more possibility to the n+1 field and the network system, so that it can execute what corresponds; This is where the magical, the extraordinary and the wonderful happen.

So, our job as human beings are to balance our Neuroakashic® potential level (levels of consciousness). This training invites you to give yourself and others the integration process, it is there where you can observe everything extraordinary and all this unimaginable that exists in the human mind.

Another purpose of Neuroakashic®, is that teachers are the best teachers, students the best students, education or health professionals, employers, professionals; By accessing and having Neuroakashic®, they can be as effective and productive in each of the areas of their life. Therefore, it is reaching all sectors and the entire population in general, so that it can have an impact on their personal, family, professional, work and general life.

Share with children, adults, pregnant women, health professionals, education professionals, individual groups, scientific, cultural, technological areas, etc. that keep us in balance, well-being and productivity to improve our quality of life. The training is designed to integrate the neural brain organization, as it progresses, we feel ready to continue in the integration process towards the great consciousness of unity.

Finally, we will observe this transformation in ourselves and that also invites the transformation to share all this with the environment, with other n+1 fields, remember that the purpose is to share and expand. What works from basic training from Akashic Activator® Unlimited Light® to Neuroakashic® Great Network System and other advanced classes?

The answer is cellular fuel.

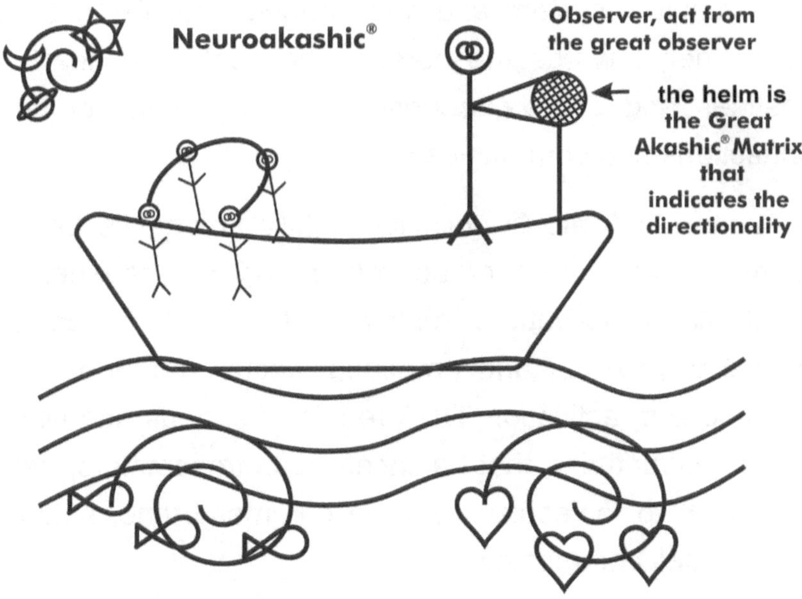

Akashic Activator® Unlimited Light®

The activator comes from the activation, the activation comes from the activator; the activator is the observer, and this is related to the control panel within neural network systems. The transformer is light, the return to essence and the integrating process of the observer and observed. Akashic activator® unlimited light® makes adjustments from micro to macro cellular level, works on the processes of neural organizational structure, which is brain plasticity, Neuroplasticity and the genome.

Then, an akashic activator® unlimited light® session works what corresponds to the network system of each user, indicating the n+1 field. This akashic activator® unlimited light® series is a series of holographic codes or patterns, the maximum expanded and amplified unlimited power of the light definition and that connects to all the switches and transmitters that are in the network system and that connect with the akashic® transformer, towards the cerebral hemispheres: heart and intestines and coccyx, connecting with millions of neural connections and communications.

Akashic activator® unlimited light® among its benefits: gamma waves, memory activation and cell regeneration, pineal gland activation, realignment, energy adjustment, release of physical and emotional toxins, immune system strengthening, activation, DNA repair, of strands and tissues, energy restructuring that balances neurotransmitters, benefit from micro to molecular from the cell membrane, balancing neuronal cell communication.

In addition, it reduces the effects of natural (cosmic radiation) and artificial radiation. It is a cell rejuvenator and prevents aging. In addition, it balances the microbiota of the intestine. Reduces the effects of natural, cosmic and artificial radiation. The latter, such as radiotherapy and chemotherapy.

It has the purpose of directing from the sound waves of the user to the great central network systems, from the neural networks or great glial cell, to the great akashic® matrix and central network system. The activator takes into account and works on all network systems where the user is involved and the consequent network systems on all time lines.

Makes neural structural adjustments, preparing for connection to the neural network system to the great akashic® matrix and from the user's network system, taking measurements and making adjustments to connect neural networks to the whole and balance the brain in high or hyper Neuroakashic® potential.

Its purpose is to connect and achieve coherence of the heart-brain, Gaia and GAM, at the cellular, DNA, neural, heart-mind-soul-spirit connection, adoption of light, network system, energy and masculine and feminine balance, it is done in person, and online, individually and in groups.

There is no observer intervention when the principles of unity are expressed during the session. It is done without expectations, since the same light that expands by itself; The session is carried out through the series, being and acting as the observer, from the great observer in the respective and corresponding n+1 fields.

In conclusion, Akashic Activator® Unlimited Light® works from birth, helping to make the encounter with yourself, since you were in your mother's womb and up to eighteen months before the union of cells to integrate and adopt the process of light in the heart. Love and photonic light flow through your cells and divine grace, understanding through love what we were created for.

In Akashic Activator® Unlimited Light® they are of the benefits that purify and cleanse blood cells. It has been perceived how adjustments are made from the blood level and how the blood transports information from other time-space realities.

Akashic Activator® II

Akashic activator® II continues to work, preparing, integrating and balancing the neuroplasticity and the processes of neurogenesis (the birth and proliferation of new neurons in the brain) and neuronal regeneration. Other benefits:

- Structural adjustments at levels: physical, mental, emotional, etc. At the level of organs, skin and in all body systems.

- Adjustments at the micro and macro cellular level, movement of photonic light at the cellular level, preparing for the Akashic Connection®.

- Cellular tissue restructuration.

- Neuroplasticity.

- Mental reset.

Akashic Connection®

Its purpose is to work on neuroplasticity and neurogenesis, to enhance neuronal activity and neuronal synapses, through the akashic connection® process. It is a process, which is in continuous work to be able to integrate and prepare for the process of balancing the Neuroakashic® potential level, which connects and balances the neural network system and the great akashic® matrix, it is the Akashic Connection® process and evolution of the brain or continuous neural evolution.

It is the prolonged synchronicity of love and light, among its benefits are: cosmic DNA activation, connecting with the whole, recoding and reconfiguring DNA, in all its facets, connection with the heart-brain-Gaia-GAM, mental reset, connection to mother earth, n+1 fields and Neuroakashic® network systems, works on neuronal regeneration (neurogenesis), anchoring to the central crystal of mother earth and connecting neural networks with the great Neuroakashic® universe, structural adjustments at the level of organs, skin and in all body systems, at all micro and macro levels, restoration and integration of the *self*, as if various parts were fragmented, united and connected in all timelines.

Neuroakashic® Connection

With the aim of developing superior abilities in people, and achieving a state of equilibrium, fullness, well-being, optimal health, coherence, multiple intelligences, high Neuroakashic® potential, among others; psychic, artistic, sports, scientific and other capacities are being developed and strengthened.

- Active neural connection.

- Modulation and activation of the glia cell.

- Splitting, integration of the *self*.

- Condensation of photonic light and activated light fields.

- Oneness with the whole.

- Integration.

Neuroakashic® Expandia

It is the controller, transport vehicle, control or information panel that transmits signals in the form of holographic patterns: images, geometric figures, codes, languages, etc; Its purpose is to move and integrate network systems: neural, family, ancestral, planetary, universal, cosmic, universes, multi-universes, and the whole. They integrate cycles and timelines, among others, preparing to join the great network system.

Jacobo Grinberg mentioned that there is a zone in the brain that contains all the information of the processor, in this case, the neural field (for us, the n+1 field) is related to the vehicle of transformations or central processor, which is for us the control panel *expandia*; the system consists of a peripheral processor that is in charge of transforming the signals, the information it collects is transformed into geometric patterns; For this reason, Grinberg sees the similarity between the system they have built and the way the portion of the human brain works. (Grinberg, 1976, pg. 60). With this, observe how the great akashic® matrix is in replicity to the brain.

Referring to the replication of the great akashic® matrix (GAM) and the brain, *expandia*, tries to balance the plasticity of GAM with the human brain, since it is, is connected to the pineal gland, cerebral hemispheres, heart, intestines, coccyx towards the central crystal of mother earth and again towards the cerebral hemispheres. *Expandia* connects and communicates from the brain and cerebral hemispheres, as a circuit connected to the rest of the human body, in the form of interconnected or interrelated networks throughout the body and hence in network connection with other brains in hyper high brain power or Neuroakashic® potential, towards great network systems and the GMA.

Among the benefits of receiving this class are: equilibrium in the levels of rootlessness and major anchorage, equilibrium of the brain potential or Neuroakashic® potential, equilibrium of the feminine and masculine principles, equilibrium of coherence and harmonic state, integration of the system and ancestral lineage. It integrates non-separation, such as the energy of money, love, other realities, among others.

Neuroakashic® Network System

The purpose is to integrate the 4th. act, become and transform in the great observer of network systems and the great akashic® matrix with which the observer bases are laid from the Akashic Activator® Unlimited Light® class to reach this class of network systems, where you are the observer acting from the great observer; you are the great observer, you are part of that great Akashic® matrix and network systems.

In this class the great observer, the integration process and the *non-separation* in the network systems are integrated.

Neuroakashic® Great Network System

In this advanced class, the observer becomes the great observer, in the balance of hyper high brain power or Neuroakashic® potential, this is the consciousness of unity. Where through superior capabilities such as advanced remote vision, observe and navigate the great network systems. In addition, it allows to develop maximum power and creative, coherent and expansive brain performance; the equilibrium of ancestral, family, universal, galactic, multi-universe network systems, the great observer, the transformation, the interaction in and from the great network system, the great unity consciousness, the n+1 fields, equilibrium, well-being, health, fullness, in a coherent, progressive, essential and creative process.

Akashic Activator® Crystals

In this n+1 field, the great observer continues to be integrated and interact with the consciousness of mother earth Gaia. The benefits it brings are, expanded remote vision and the relationship with expanded brains in network connection. Crystals function as vehicles and signal amplifiers for the n+1 fields, in the neural network systems, within this n+1 field, gamma waves have benefits.

Learning is achieved through four sessions from the n+1 field, akashic activator® crystals, using crystals, quartz, gems, stones, etc. as a vehicle. This can be taken in person or online, group and individual applied to children, youth and adults: akashic activator® crystals, remote vision, n+1 fields, individual and group.

This, is the explanation of the use of crystals as a vehicle in the field, it happens that when an object acts as a vehicle in the n+1 field, the vehicles in the n+1 fields can alter the structure of the interrelated network systems of the great akashic® matrix, therefore, decodable interference patterns are produced by the control panel or *Expandia* information panel.

Akashic Activator® Prenatal & Birthing

Students within the Neuroakashic® program have been observed in the postpartum, maternity and birth process of their babies. There is a balance, neural effect in and from pregnant women and babies as a result of Neuroakashic® sessions or classes, either online or in person.

We carried out a study with boys and girls born within the n+1 fields of Neuroakashic®, the result showed that they are emotionally and mentally more balanced boys and girls, with highly advanced skills and talents, with the remote vision capacity of the observer and the equilibrium in the Neuroakashic® potential level, their neural connection, evolved and advanced remote vision, balanced, healthy, healthful, intelligent, with very advanced gifts, abilities and potentialities, with a lot of wisdom and intelligence, they are leaders, with a firm character in their decisions, friendly, observant, they honor the elements of water, air, earth and fire, just as they love the moon, they have a good relationship with animals, they are playful, observers, loving and knowledgeable.

In this class, we work from the various n+1 fields for prenatal, perinatal, birth and postnatal study. Among its benefits of receiving this class: accompaniment and containment for the mother and baby pre and postpartum, preparation for delivery and birth of the baby, prenatal and post-natal development.

Akashic Activator® Kids

The purpose of this n+1 field, of this class, is to integrate areas of language, learning, mental and emotional containment, among others. Furthermore, they can balance their Neuroakashic® potential and integrate all their superior abilities, high capacities and multiple intelligences. It works with a specialized methodology for children; to integrate all the benefits of this class, from the benefits of gamma waves, which help children achieve a equanimous, balanced and harmonic state, remote vision, strengthens the immune system, regulates metabolism, regenerates cells, activates memory and repairs cell tissues, repairs DNA.

Akashic Activator® Musical

This class has the purpose of integrating sound frequencies in hertz, accessing this n+1 field, using as vehicles the various musical instruments, such as bowls, gong, bells, drums, guitar, piano, violin, among others; receiving the benefit of music is the set of sounds that is anchored to the field.

The light is sound and it reads the vibration and frequency of the field, it leads the way to correct, harmonize, restructure and adjust the said field. In some occasions, the sound is defragmented into words and grouped into bands 1 and 2, 3 series of 3 and integrated into space-time, in addition, they are located and focused at some point in the network systems.

Akashic Activator® Business

This class works from this n+1 field, with the aim of knowing how the brain and neural network systems work; Regardless of whatever area or profession you are in, today it is important to know and practice it. The observer participant will be able to integrate psychosocial risk factors, as well as promote a favorable organizational environment in the workplace.

This n+1 field, favors business connection and teamwork, contributes something *more* than anyone else has seen, probably to the collective conscience, which is the directionality of the community to be in direct relationship, or the network connection to something else bigger. The observer is required to integrate risk aversion and fear, since the n+1 fields of businesses, companies and / or corporations are ready to access them in their harmonious state; they are human networks that are in the continuous, coherent and progressive process to integrate into something bigger. The purpose of the consciousness leader is to see the world as a network that everything is connected to everything without separation and that forms a network with the vehicle of giving and sharing.

Akashic Activator® Places

Its purpose is to access this field and carry out studies to places such as: houses, buildings, land, among others. The benefits of receiving an akashic activator® places session are: integration, well-being, balance of the n+1 field: house, land, building, etc. to transform into abundant and prosperous places, it improves the physical, mental and emotional health of the owners, inhabitants and visitors. The first akashic activator® places matrix session, is the energy, matter, protons, neutrons, electrons of the place. The second session of akashic activator® places n+1 field, are the neurons of the place and the third session of akashic activator® place networks, is the set of all the interrelated neurons of the place.

Akashic Activator® Animals

This n+1 field provides a direct connection with animals and a relationship with nature, where the manifestation of animals enters the total connection with mother earth. Each animal fertilizes the field, animals help us to be in unity connection with the whole. In addition to the benefits, they provide us with the balance of neurotransmitters and the cerebral hemispheres. Remember that animals have Neuroakashic® potential, this class will help them to be in well-being and fullness.

Neuroakashic® Business

In this class from this n+1 field, the purpose of Neuroakashic® business is to prepare the user to become the consciousness leader, an effective, efficient and productive negotiator and mediator, so that he can achieve coherent, progressive and successful negotiations. Thus, achieving lasting, measurable and impeccable effects and results. In addition, facilitating the user to increase the level of consciousness of the environment that surrounds him, as how it benefits or affects his interaction with it, through the identification and knowledge of the n+1 fields.

Teach the negotiator to integrate the strategies and abilities of negotiation and communication in the n+1 fields, under the principles of unity in a continuous, integrated and expanded process. Knowledge of the n+1 fields is taught, from the beginning to the end of the negotiation and of the network systems to know and locate the components and elements of the field, circumstances, events, people, etc.

Likewise, holographically placing information in the n+1 field, in this case the solution is anchored in the n+1 field within the simulation of the interactive n+1 field. The n+1 field is knowledge and interaction with the environment in general and with the respective network systems, to holographically impact the results of the negotiation.

Throughout the development of this class, you will be able to improve your skills of mental and emotional containment, handling of emotions and empathy in negotiation; as well as the construction of agreements from the principles of unity, to be a consciousness leader and an expert negotiator, coherent and conscious. It will be necessary to anchor to the field, the solution and the negotiation of the conflict, to finish the negotiation equanimous and with directionality from the network connection to the unit.

Neuroakashic® Crystals

In this advanced class, n+1 field is accessed, brain power or Neuroakashic® potential is balanced to reach the hyper high level, which is the new consciousness, the unity consciousness, the new reality, the new creation of fields n+1, the integration of the great network system.

New educational model

In this book, a new comprehensive educational model corresponding to this new era is proposed, a creative and collaborative education, based on principles of unity, as a team that can provide solutions to conflicts and problems. This educational model is based on competency standards, which are the set of knowledge, abilities, skills and attitudes that a person must have to carry out a work activity, with a high level of performance.

In addition, this Neuroakashic® educational model is based on socio-emotional competences as indicated by the Organization for Economic Development Cooperation (OEDC) on its page. In the model of social and emotional skills, its guiding axes should include the characteristics of: collaboration, open mind, engaging with others, emotional regulation, performance of abilities, among which are: sociability, assertiveness, tolerance, creativity, empathy, cooperation, trust, control of emotions and resistance to stress, responsibility, motivation, self-control, among others.

In a continuous learning process, to achieve the integration of multiple intelligences and achieve balance, well-being and productivity, which integrates skills and high abilities with flexible, effective and durable tools, in a conscious, continuous, coherent, progressive and expansive teaching process, to achieve unity consciousness, through containment tools and didactic techniques.

Neuroakashic®, is a comprehensive educational model, is adaptable and self-sustainable, it integrates some aspects of the SOLVE methodology from the perspective of gender equality and confidentiality, in order to implement policies and actions to promote health in individuals, at work, family and link the environment, the community and other institutions.

Jacobo Grinberg, in his book "conscious brain", mentions

that the educational work of our era should consist of finding techniques for decoding the akashic record, rather than transmitting specific information. Our children should learn the use and handling of these techniques in order to pass through the knowledge contained in space-time. This is the reason of the existence of this Neuroakashic® model.

Grinberg also mentioned that geometric schemes, visual images, codes, when viewed, activate a brain state that serves to activate a neuronal field. (Grinberg, 1991, pg. 80). Our model is based on holographic patterns, interactively through Neuroakashic® cellular fuels, such as the new education proposal, which the educational system should promote for the development of images, as a basis for the acquisition of knowledge.

We propose a methodology that integrates and forms the new educational model for children and adults; the new creative and unity education, so that the corresponding solutions are solved effectively and assertively as a team. Thus, in this book, it presents a Neuroakashic® educational model, which integrates skills and high capacities from a true consciousness leader, with flexible, effective and lasting tools, in a conscious, continuous, coherent, progressive and expansive teaching process to achieve unity consciousness. Through emotional and mental containment tools, didactic techniques, in a continuous learning process and the development of competences to achieve integration, balance, well-being and productivity.

Through three axes and virtual continuing education, the Neuroakashic® program offers us an online E-learning platform, conferences, master class and congresses. We are sharing the

Neuroakashic® channel, to share and expand internationally. The second axis is the creation of virtual and face-to-face theme parks, the last axis is the creation of virtual or in person campuses, cities and Neuroakashic® communities.

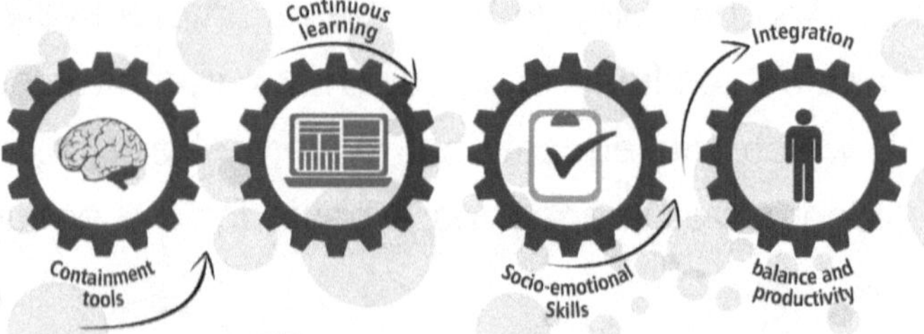

Conclusion

The process of raising consciousness is a substantial health issue today, where the importance of our mental health is vital; From these principles, Neuroakashic® emerges as a new comprehensive educational model, providing benefits such as emotional and mental containment, in attention to psychosocial factors, of our mission, which is to share and expand day by day.

The purpose is to become consciousness leader. The truth is the step, the process in which the light is defined, the step between what separates towards unity, is to let the truth enter the heart, what you are currently living is the step before integrating non-separation. This non-separation has to do with the neuronal wiring, since it forms a new neural cell network in the brain, this is the process of non-separation, it does not have to do with divine actors but with integrating the principle of non-separation through the Neuroakashic® neural fuels.

Today we have the transformation tool in neural network systems and towards the great network in networks system. You can measure and check the level or degree and the existence of consciousness through Neuroakashic® through some factors such as: the theory of n+1 fields, oxygen levels in the blood, heart rate, the measurement of levels of rootlessness and greater anchorage, this last ones represent the measure of the degrees or levels of consciousness; the relationship and the confirmation that we are part of a great network system in network connection with other brains and the existence of the hyper high brain potential or Neuroakashic® potential, that is, the hyper harmonic state, hyper high coherence of the heart-brain, the full equilibrium, the super or supra consciousness, the consciousness of unity. Neuroakashic® is replicable and all that replicates is science.

Currently the neuronal brain advance that exists has advanced in terms of knowledge. Neuroakashic® allows us to be better human beings, endowed with all the superior abilities and capacities, allowing us create new n+1 fields to form a great new network system, for the well-being, love and equilibrium of all humanity.

Therefore, we are ready to share this new comprehensive educational model, which aims to become shared and expanded nationally and internationally in schools, private and public institutions, companies, businesses, corporations, organizations, areas of health, security, among others.

We can say that one of the missions is to convert and achieve through this knowledge, to be the best human beings, best people, to find love and to live in unity, honoring each other. Everything is already, there is no expectation, where everything and nothing is, where there is no place for judgment, expectation more than love and truth. Connect and work our own evolution process, wherever there is in the heart as a seat to reconnect with our origin, own love and light that is in the heart, where there is no intervention, love and truth are manifested during the connection.

Neuroakashic®, the great observer is our heart, it is the heart of the mother earth Gaia, the purpose is to generate awareness of love in you, in the generosity of your heart. It does not matter the settings, the people, the roles, etc. when love is already within each one, expanded and amplified. Allow ourselves to be and act from the great observer, integrate and work every day the principles of unity to achieve our own balance.

If your relationship with money responds to your relationship with light, the energy of money is unlimited; things do not have to have intention, it is enough to observe that the process of the great observer is carried out, so that it materializes in the n+1 field, rather than the intention itself.

The principle of giving is the engine for creating something bigger and giving it continuity in neural network systems. In the principle of giving, Neuroakashic® is integrated to balance brain potential and provide solutions to some diseases. Likewise, it gives way to the creation of new sciences, new n+1 fields, new laws, a new era of integration and a new medicine, which will allow the integration of family network systems.

Finding ourselves is our daily task, as well as strengthening our connection with love and integrating the non-separation between the observer and the observed. What is light? The light is knowing that there is nothing more than: you and the light, the light is you, result: the one, the uniqueness and the understanding are the light. Know that, within the integration process, the strand, the photonic light gene and the twelfth strand in our DNA that connects us with our own light, is already in us, what we have always been, what we are and what we will be.

Medicine as we know it today, is going to change to the new medicine, science will jump to the great transformation to give rise to new sciences, new laws; the cycles of life and death will be as one, without separation, since death is flying in the network. The awakening of consciousness is the great observer, the consciousness of unity is inevitable; as a whole as unity consciousness, the earth's electromagnetic field is moving.

What it defines is the high or hyper high level, which works in the transforming language in neural networks and performs the modulating effect, anchoring itself to the n+1 field and achieving results. The user, has the purpose of consciousness to achieve deeper and unimaginable effects that may exist. The brain sees an opportunity where others do not visibly see it. Money is light and therefore it is unlimited, it will never end, things depend on how you see them, so reality can be perceived differently, due to the Neuroakashic® level of consciousness. The ability to get ahead is resilience, which is seeing the light where there is chaos.

The secret is to let be, observe and trust that something bigger accommodates and adjusts, what corresponds for each one in the respective and corresponding network system, without forcing and worrying about absolutely nothing, observing without judgment and without expectation, through the eyes of light, and of the love that is the force of creation and the motor of life itself. Reaching love, from now on it will be your great internal mastery.

It is the hyper high potential, it is what you have always sought, and it is to live fully in unity consciousness. The human being is love, without separation that is the magnificent and magnificent creative force within his heart. You are the great network that integrates the network systems, they are also all the family systems, the system of ancestral lineage, male and female. Understand that sometimes, to advance in our evolution process, people are and others are not, and it is normal, observe and develop the capacity of the observer.

The aim is to create, generate and integrate unity consciousness from education, to restructure the social tissue and integrate families into network systems, giving rise to father, mother and integrating the whole. Allow you to observe and integrate the principles of unity and share boys, girls, women, men and families, in various areas such as health, education of children and adults for the formation and integration of families.

The way of doing business has already been transformed, since the relationship with the principle of giving and our environment changed into a new transformation of giving in human relationships. Learn and integrate the principles of unity in businesses, companies, organizations and corporations. Become consciousness leader by putting your talents, gifts and abilities at the service of others. Give, share and expand.

Caring for our planet, working for justice and peace, conforming ourselves as self-sustaining cities, from the perspective of gender, equality, parity and achieving well-being, balance and health; retake the principles of unity and achieve greater consciousness through Neuroakashic® training. It will be necessary to maintain the balance of the n+1 fields, in the network systems and the great akashic® matrix to achieve the hyper high Neuroakashic® potential, this is the foundation and next step to the unification of reality.

Cultivate your faith, commit to the process and everything will be given, because wonderful things will happen, open your heart, open your mind, the message is for everyone. It is time to recognize the present moment and treasure what is being lived today, without feeling that we carry. A practitioner shares and expands light; A facilitator transmits, lives, experiments and expands unity consciousness. Dare to live them.

The person is not the one who decides what to take from the field, it is the field itself that decides and puts what the great observer requires, since he is wise and intelligent. There is nothing to worry about, that tomorrow will worry about itself. There is no plan, there is no way, because you are the plan, you are the way, you are the great observer. So, our purpose is to transmit Neuroakashic® fuels to integrate the principles of unity and put them at the service of the field; in other words, fertilizing the field is balancing our brain power, our Neuroakashic® potential.

As I conclude this book, I would like to remind all my readers that learning to see our own world, without judgment or expectation, helps us transform our own world; previous experiences help us to be the best humans today. Being *the great observer* of your own life is freedom, it is allowing you to observe the extraordinary, to achieve more organized, supportive, creative, collaborative, full and expansive societies, cities and communities of knowledge. Next, a poem of my authorship, inspired by the light, your light.

Light poem

And if in every act of love there is light,

the consequence is the same,

your human act towards the light is already,

the light is working in you,

I see you with the same love

which the light would see you with,

the missing piece was you,

my lesson is to see the light,

and I found the light in my actions

when I was looking for someone else,

the light was there

experience love without separation

like you see your partner that is your relationship with light.

We honor our work and that of our ancestors. May your teachings be imparted by all mankind! May it reach every corner of every nation!

The light is already in me, the light is already in you, the light is already in us!

Glossary

ABC of the observer: refers to the integration of the steps to achieve the understanding of the great observer.

Assemblage point: refers to the emanations that exert outside and inside the cocoon or luminous egg: it is what makes it possible to perceive and in turn.

Biohematic: refers to the union of two words bio, life and blood hematic, which is the life of blood; for us it is the catalyst and motor that purifies the cells in the blood.

Completeness: refers to the act of totality.

Demystifying light: it reduces the mystical or supernatural that is attributed to light and shows with real events what is considered remote from reality.

Delta, Theta, Alpha, Beta and Gamma: brain waves are considered to be the electrical activity produced by the brain; they are divided into 5 waves that indicate the state of the brain's functioning.

Disruptive: term in English that refers to change.

DMT: Dimethyltryptamine, a chemical substance, also called the divine particle that connects to something greater, has an intrinsic relationship with the crystals of time and provides the ability to observe the various realities in the lines and cycles of space-time.

DNA: is deoxyribonucleic acid, a protein found in the core of cells and constitutes the main component of the genetic material of living beings.

Emotio: refers to the feeling of the word emotion in Latin.

Expandia: refers to the term that designates a machine, also called the control panel or the information contained in network systems.

Field n+1: is the way to call your electromagnetic field, the field of another person, the neuronal field, the field of your house, city, state, country, planet and world, and the sum of these is field n+1.

Gaia: refers to planet earth.

GAM: it is one of the ways in which we can call the great akashic® matrix, the same machinery that contains all network systems.

Glia cells: They are part of the nervous system. In the brain, the glia cells can control the survival of neurons. They play a key role in the development of neurological diseases.

Hyperneurons: or also called mother neurons of our planet earth Gaia, which are connected with our cerebral hemispheres, heart, intestines, coccyx and made the central crystal of mother earth.

Meissner effect: This refers to when a magnet levitates or when it is placed on a superconducting material.

Memory of the future: refers to the meaning of traveling through time or network systems.

Neuroplasticity: it is the capacity and potential of the nervous system to mold itself and form new nervous connections.

Polymath: refers to a person who has all the knowledge or wisdom and is synonymous of superior abilities or high abilities.

Schumman resonances: refer to the heartbeat or heart of our planet earth, it is the indicator or meter of the earth's magnetic field.

SOLVE: is the methodology of the International Labor Organization (ILO), which integrates health promotion with the policy of safety and health at work. Contributes to the prevention of psychosocial risks and well-being in the workplace; It has 9 guiding axes: stress, economic stress, HIV, nutrition, healthy sleep, alcohol and drugs, tobacco, physical activity and violence.

Bibliography

- Paolelli, E. (2014). *The new frontier of neuroscience.* Italy: Nuova Ipsa Editore.

- Braden, G. (2007). *The divine matrix: a bridge between time, space, beliefs and miracles.* 2nd. Edition. Mexico: Editorial Sirio. United States: Hay House.

- Pribram H. and J. Martín Ramírez. (1980). *Brain Mind and Hologram;* 1st. Edition. Spain: Editorial Alhambra S.A.

- Grinberg, J. (1988). *Psychophysiology of power.* 1st. Edition. México D.F.: National Institute for the Study of Consciousness.

- Grinberg, J. (2008). *Flow in without me.* 1st. Edition. México, D.F: Ediciones B México, S.A de C.V.

- Fuster, M. (2015). *Neuroscience; the brain foundations of our freedom.* México D.F.: Ediciones Culturales Paidós, S.A. de C.V.

- Grinberg, J. (1991). *Sintergic Theory.* 1st. Edition. México D.F.: INPEC.

- Grinberg, J. (1976). *The vehicle of transformations.* 1st. edition. México, D.F.: Editorial trillas.

- Dispensa, J. (2008). *Develop your brain, the science to change the mind,* Buenos Aires, Argentina: Editorial Kier S.A., 1ª. Edition.

- Marín, G. (1999). *To read Carlos Castañeda.* 2nd. Edition, Mexico, D.F.: Colofón, S.A.

- Grinberg, J. (1979). *The* conscious brain, psychophysiology of consciousness 2. 1st. Edition. Mexico: Editorial Trillas.

- Attie Leah B. y Valle, A. (2017). <u>*Alice in the country of conscience, about Grinberg and her disappearance*</u>. Mexico: Lunaria Ediciones.

- Mc Taggart, L. (2007). *The Field.* 2nd. Edition. Spain: Editorial Sirio, S.A.

- Lipton, Bruce; *The biology of belief. 1st. International Latin American Conference.* Buenos Aires, Argentina. www.creandotuvida.com

- Dr. Ryke Geerd Hamer- *The origin of evil (cancer)* (TVE 1995) complete. Recovered from: https://m.youtube.com/watch?v=x3jVN5-UVRs

- Sciotto, E. and Niripil, E. Brain waves, consciousness and cognition. *Organization for the prevention and promotion of health in education.* Recovered from: https://www.academia.edu/35611100/ONDAS_CEREBRALES_CONCIENCIA_Y_COGNICION

- Martinelli, A. *Nikola Tesla and his journey through time: "I saw the past, the present and the future at the same time.* Recovered from: https://youtu.be/nA44945OGgc

- Mather, T. (2018). *How heart rate variability affects emotion regulation brain networks.* Recovered from: Curr Opin Behav Sci.Doi: 10.106 / j.cobeha.2017.12.017

- Fuster, J. (s.f.). Networks110: The soul is in the network of the brain, neuroscience. Recovered from: https://www.youtube.com/watch?v=jgTH2Sb5pys

- Saadoun, Angeline, (s.f.); *the existence of time crystals is confirmed, a new state of matter;* Recovered from: https://www.vix.com/es/ciencia/177359/la-ciencia-descubrio-que-los-rasgos-de-nuestro-rostro-tienen-esta-increible-relacion-con-nuestro?utm_source = next_article

- Social and emotional education. (s.f.). Recovered from: https://www.oecd.org/education/ceri/study-on-social-and-emotional-skills-the-study.htm

- Global coherence research; retrieved from: https://www.heartmath.org/gci/research/global-coherence/

- https://www.ilo.org/safework/info/instr/WCSM_203117/lang--es/index.htm

- https://definicion.de/desmitificar/

- https://es.m.wikipedia.org/wiki/Dimetiltriptamina

- Castellano López Bernardo & Berta González de Mingo. Neuroscience, mind and brain. Research and Science. Retrieved from: https: //www.investigationyciencia.es/revistas/mente-y-cerebro/emociones-musicales-402/clulas-gliales-4479. July / August 2005.

Akashic School®

Neuroakashic® International Certification

By Akashic School Inc

Online or in person

1) Akashic Activator ® Unlimited Light ®, Practitioner

2) Akashic Activator® II Practitioner

3) Akashic Connection® Practitioner

4) Akashic Activator ® Unlimited Light ® Facilitator

5) Akashic Activator® II Facilitator

6) Akashic Connection® Facilitator

7) Neuroakashic® Connection Practitioner

8) Neuroakashic® Expandia Practitioner

9) Neuroakashic® Network System Practitioner

10) Neuroakashic® Great Network System Practitioner

11) Neuroakashic® Connection Facilitator

12) Neuroakashic® Expandia Facilitator

13) Neuroakashic® Network System Facilitator

14) Neuroakashic® Great Network System Facilitator

Advanced classes, Practitioner & Facilitator:

- Akashic Activator® Dance
- Akashic Activator® Musical
- Akashic Activator® Oratory
- Akashic Activator® Crystals
- Akashic Activator® Writers
- Akashic Activator® Business
- Akashic Activator® Animals
- Akashic Activator® Children
- Akashic Activator® Places
- Akashic Activator® Prenatal & Birthing
- 4 days, Field (n+1)
- 3 days, Neuroakashic® Business
- 3 days, Neuroakashic® Crystals
- 2 days, Love Relationships
- 2 days, Cycles of time
- 2 days, Money and You

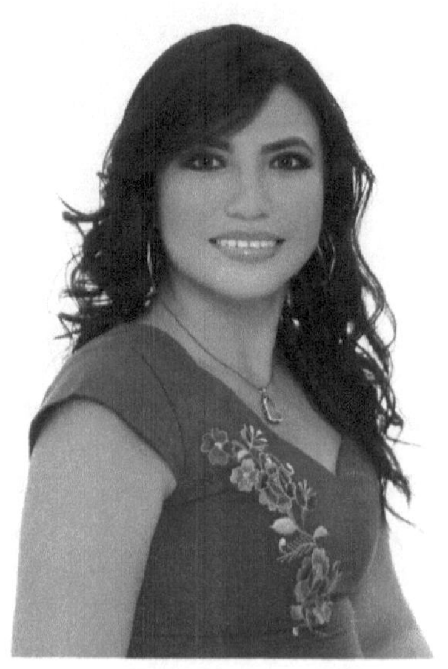

More info:

Contact the author and learn more at:

www.neuroakashic.us

www.escuelaakashica.com

neuroakashic@hotmail.com

FB: /AnaSilviaNeuroAkashic

YT: Ana Silvia Lara

IG: ana_silvia_neuro_akashico

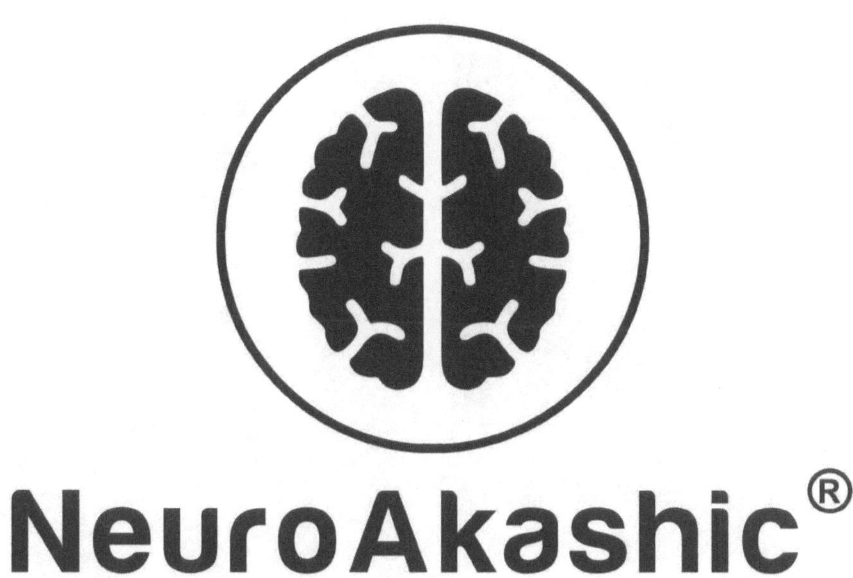